MW01435074

THE COMPLETE COOKBOOK ON THE PALEO DIET SPECIAL BREAKFASTS 2021/22

The Complete Guide on the Paleo Diet with all the recipes on Breakfasts, a way to lose weight starting in the morning, if you love morning breakfasts this is the book for you.

Erika Lombardi

ERIKA LOMBARDI

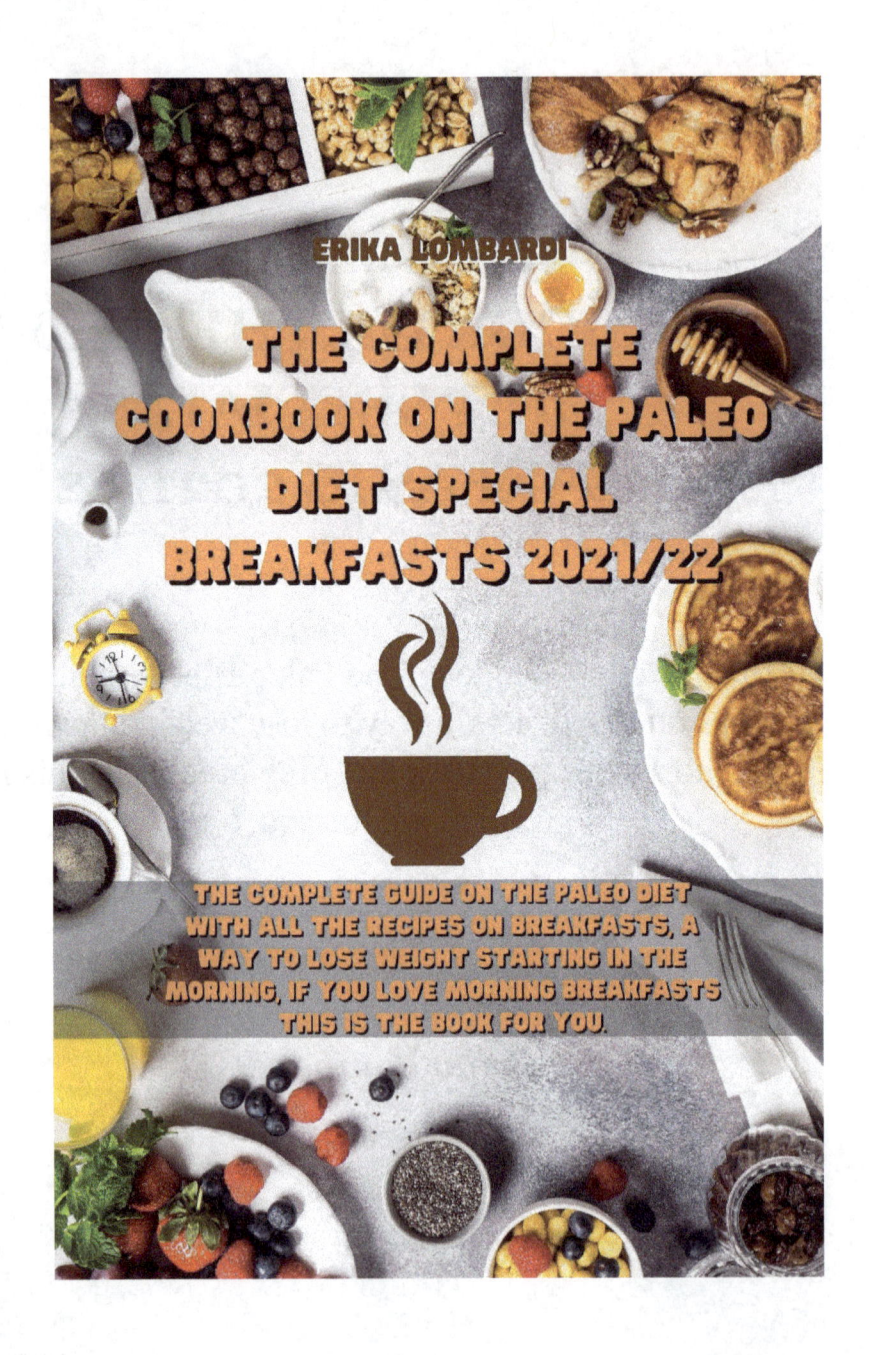

THE COMPLETE COOKBOOK ON THE PALEO DIET SPECIAL BREAKFASTS 2021/22

THE COMPLETE GUIDE ON THE PALEO DIET WITH ALL THE RECIPES ON BREAKFASTS, A WAY TO LOSE WEIGHT STARTING IN THE MORNING, IF YOU LOVE MORNING BREAKFASTS THIS IS THE BOOK FOR YOU.

Table Of Contents

INTRODUCTION 12

BREAKFAST 16

HEALTHY BREAKFAST BURRITO PALEO STYLE 17

BREAKFAST PALEO CASSEROLE 20

SCRAMBLED EGGS WITH ONIONS, MUSHROOM AND TOMATO 23

BAKED PROSCIUTTO CUPS 26

FRUIT SALAD BREAKFAST 29

ALMOND PANCAKES 32

SHRIMP OMELETTE WITH AVOCADO 35

ALMOND CHURROS WAFFLES 38

VEGETABLE WITH HARDBOILED EGGS AND HAM 41

LOADED APRICOT SQUARES 44

BREAKFAST SAUSAGE WITH MASHED "POTATO" 47

EGGS BENEDICT 50

STUFFED PALEO BAGUETTE 53

POTATO PANCAKES 56

HAM AND EGGS WITH POTATO 59

MINCED PORK ON FRIED EGG 62

NUTTY FRENCH TOAST 65

RAISIN BREAD WITH CINNAMON 68

EGGPLANT WITH EGG 71

GREEN-EYED SMOOTHIE 74

CHOCOLATE BANANA PANCAKE 77

BREAKFAST SAUSAGE PATTY 80

PALEO GRANOLA 83

BEEF PATTIES WITH FENNEL 86

SALMON FILLETS WITH ALMOND MEAL 89

CHICKEN IN A BLANKET 92

FRUITY CHICKEN 95

TUNA IN MUSHROOM CAPS 98

SALMON AND CAPER SALAD WITH LEMON 101

OYSTER OMELETTE 104

SAUSAGE, BACON AND EGG BREAKFAST 107

POTATO AND MUSHROOM MEDLEY 110

DRIED CHERRY-SAGE SCOTH EGGS 113

EGGS SHAKSHUKA 116

TROUT WITH SHOESTRING SWEET POTATOES 119

DATE SHAKES 123

APPLE-FLACK JACKS 126

RASPERRY BANANA SORBET 129

FRESH FRUIT 'N SPINACH SMOOTHIE 132

HONEY GLAZED PUMPKIN DONUTS 135

SMOKED SALMON FRITTATA	138
VANILLA BERRY CREPES	141
CHOCO BANANA MUFFINS	144
TURKEY VEGGIE MEATZA	147
CARROT WALNUTS SOUFFLÉ	150
GRAIN-FREE GRANOLA	153
CONCLUSIONS	157

© Copyright 2021 by Erika Lombardi - All rights reserved.

The following Book is reproduced below with the goal of providing information that is as accurate and reliable as possible. Regardless, purchasing this Book can be seen as consent to the fact that both the publisher and the author of this book are in no way experts on the topics discussed within and that any recommendations or suggestions that are made herein are for entertainment purposes only. Professionals should be consulted as needed prior to undertaking any of the action endorsed herein.

This declaration is deemed fair and valid by both the American Bar Association and the Committee of Publishers Association and is legally binding throughout the United States.

Furthermore, the transmission, duplication, or reproduction of any of the following work including specific information will be considered an illegal act irrespective of if it is done electronically or in print. This extends to creating a secondary or tertiary copy of the work or a recorded copy and is only allowed with the express written consent from the Publisher. All additional right reserved.

The information in the following pages is broadly considered a truthful and accurate account of facts and as such, any inattention, use, or misuse of the information in question by the reader will render any resulting actions solely under their purview. There are no scenarios in which the publisher or the original author of this work can be in any fashion deemed liable for any hardship or damages that may befall them after undertaking information described herein.

Additionally, the information in the following pages is intended only for informational purposes and should thus be thought of as universal. As befitting its nature, it is presented without assurance regarding its prolonged validity or interim quality. Trademarks that are mentioned are done without written consent and can in no way be considered an endorsement from the trademark holder.

☆ *55% OFF for BookStore NOW at $ 30,95 instead of $ 41,95!* ☆

We know, in the morning we usually get up hungry and we agree that breakfast is the most important meal of the day, well if you love breakfast this is the book for you I have associated the Paleo Diet by creating the tastiest breakfasts, read to start the day with the maximum of your energy ... try to believe.

Buy is NOW and let your Customers get addicted to this amazing book!

Introduction

Paleo Breakfast - When you decide to start following the paleo diet, or as some call it, the paleontological diet, one of the first questions you ask yourself is "what can I eat?" and especially what do I eat for breakfast?

How to have a Paleo breakfast

In this article we want to answer this question by giving a series of suggestions on examples that can be very useful for those who want to start to seriously follow the paleo diet. You have to say goodbye to the classic breakfast "brioche and cappuccino" or "coffee and croissant," making way for the best foods according to the current paleo diet.

The first thing you need to do, it is now known, is to detoxify from sugar, and to do this, you can experiment with many different foods:

- An omelet with mushroom salad;
- A fruit smoothie (without sugar) with added kefir or alternatively coconut milk;
- Wild salmon with fennel salad and raspberries;
- A mix of berries and nuts;
- A glass of almond milk accompanied by macadamia nuts and dates;

For those who love cooking, it would be interesting to try also avocado pancakes (80 gr. of ripe avocado pulp, 2 eggs, 25 gr. of coconut flour, 1 tablespoon of lemon juice, 3 tablespoons of coconut milk), or chestnuts crepes or a classic paleo breakfast.

We must always be careful also to the signals that our body naturally sends us when we eat something that is not good for us: if you happen to have some disorders (mouth ulcers, rashes, the air in the stomach, constipation, ...).

Going to give instead of the basic guidelines for a proper breakfast, just remember what the dictates of the paleo diet are: our body has not yet evolved to the point of digesting well cereals, legumes, dairy products, and refined sugars, for this reason, baked goods, based on refined flours and simple carbohydrates lead us to a bad diet, irritation of the intestine and modification of the intestinal walls.

Modified intestinal walls due to these "unhealthy" foods mean that nutrients are not absorbed properly, with negative consequences, including celiac disease, obesity, and other diseases that have been developing faster and faster in recent years, thanks to the industries that offer baked goods and "various snacks," products with a "long shelf life" and easy to transport.

Thanks to the paleo diet, instead, it is possible to learn what foods are potentially harmful to our body and understand how to react when our body sends us signals of "alert" about what we are eating.

By the way, did you know that the paleo diet can also help you pass the so-called nervous hunger and give you more energy?

In short, even at breakfast, the foods to avoid are cereals (including quinoa, amaranth, buckwheat, and chia seeds), legumes, sugars (including those in soft drinks), dairy products, and especially hydrogenated fats.

Also, remember that those who have autoimmune diseases should talk to a doctor or specialized nutritionist before embarking on a paleo path.

The typical Paleo diet dish should be composed of two-thirds of plant foods and one-third of animal foods: to complete the meal, always add healthy fats that can come from avocado, extra virgin olive oil, walnuts, almonds, or virgin coconut oil.

In this cookbook, I have prepared for you a series of recipes with an avalanche of breakfasts of all tastes, and I am sure I will be able to satisfy any palate.

So let's get started!

BREAKFAST

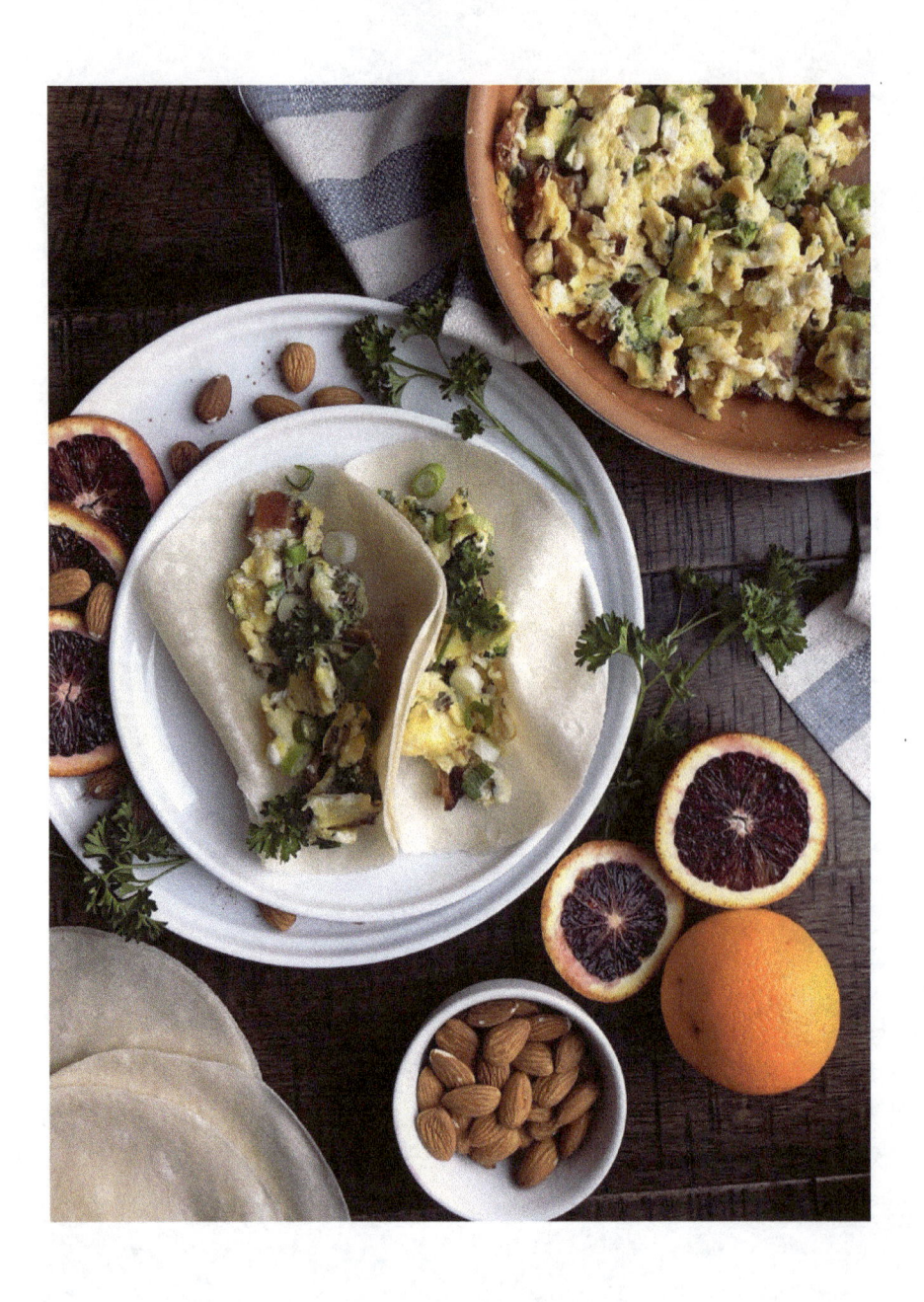

Healthy Breakfast Burrito Paleo Style

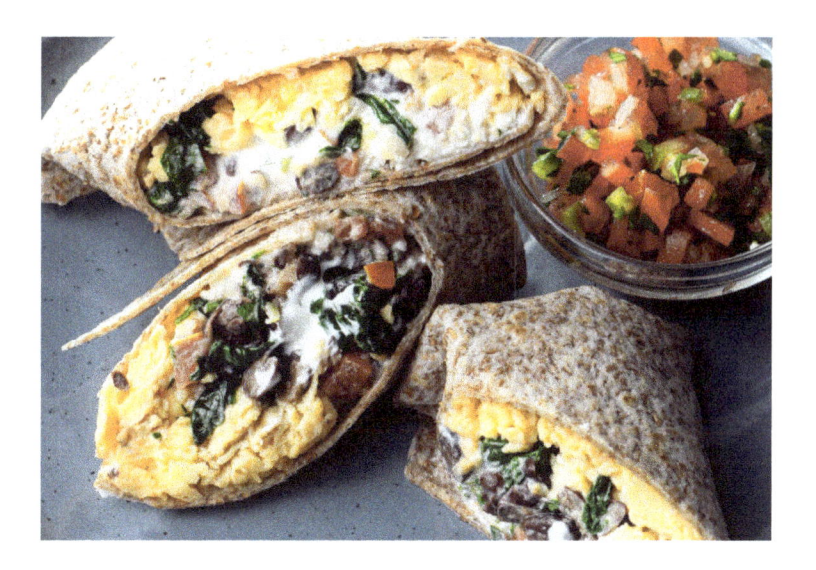

Cooking Time: 14 minutes
Servings: 3
Ingredients:

Sliced Ham
Three eggs (or egg whites)
1/2 cup chopped veggies

Directions:

Brown the chopped vegetables in a pan in a little oil.

While the vegetables cook for a few minutes, beat the eggs in a bowl and pour over the sautéed vegetables. Stir well until cooked through.

Lay out a slice of ham and place some of the vegetables in the center.

Roll the ham around the vegetable and egg mixture, then brown the ham on the skillet.

Breakfast Paleo Casserole

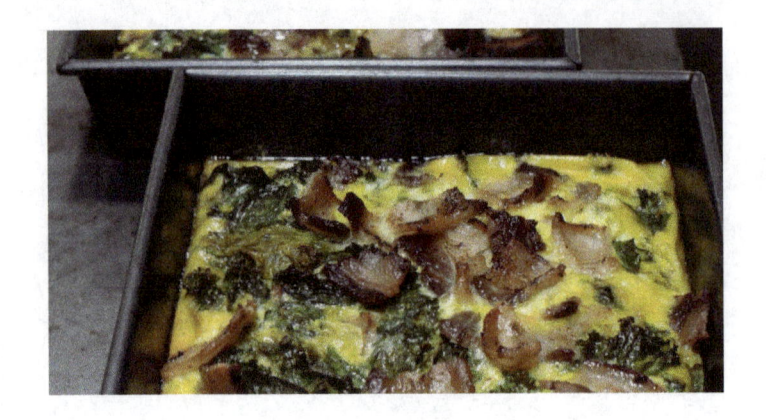

Cooking Time: 30 minutes
Servings: 8
Ingredients:

1 pound sausage
1 large sweet potato; diced
2 cups baby spinach, roughly chopped
2 large tomatoes, thinly sliced
1 green onion, diced
10 large eggs
salt and pepper to taste

Directions:

Preheat oven to about 375 degrees. Grease a glass baking dish (9x13).

Remove casings from sausage and prepare vegetables for sautéing.

Cook the sausage well for a few minutes in a large skillet, then remove it and set the sausage fat aside.

Cook the diced sweet potatoes in the sausage fat for about 10 minutes.

Mix the cooked sweet potatoes, green onions, spinach, and sausage well in a bowl.

Spread the mixture evenly over the bottom of the glass baking dish.

Beat all the eggs in a large bowl and pour evenly over the sausage and vegetable mixture.

Place the thinly sliced tomatoes on top of the mixture.

Bake in the oven for about 25 minutes.

Scrambled Eggs with Onions, Mushroom and Tomato

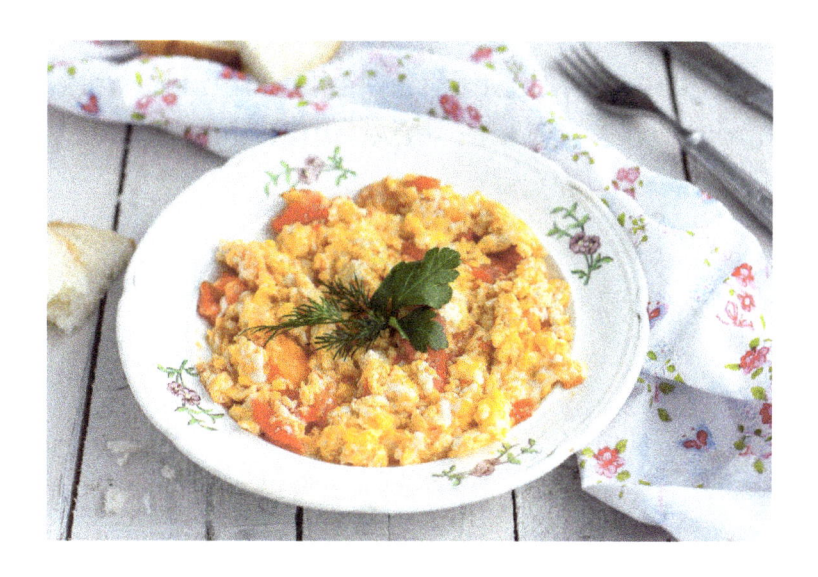

Cooking Time: 10 minutes
Servings: 2
Ingredients:

4 large eggs
3 spring onions, chopped
1/2 cup chopped mushrooms
1/2 cup chopped tomatoes
1 cup cubed ham

Directions:

Saute the chopped spring onions, mushrooms, tomatoes and ham and cook well until the ham is browned.
Break eggs over the mixture and scramble well.
Remove from pan and serve immediately.

Baked Prosciutto Cups

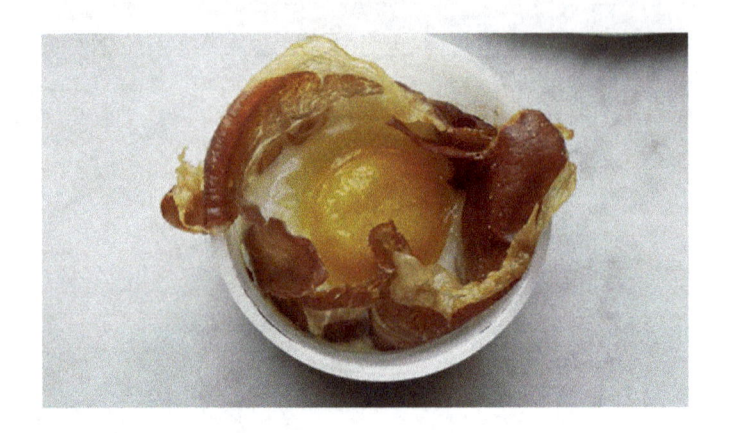

Cooking Time: 25 minutes
Servings: 1
Ingredients:

1 slice of Prosciutto
1 egg
Pepper to taste

Directions:

The oven should be preheated to 360 degrees.
Use 1 slice of prosciutto to line a ramekin or a baking tin. The prosciutto should cover the sides and bottom of the container, especially for baking tins where the egg will stick.
Crack the egg into the prosciutto cup.

Sprinkle pepper to taste.
Placed ramekin or baking tins on a tray and place in oven.
Bake for 15-20 minutes.
When done, allow standing for a few minutes.

Fruit Salad Breakfast

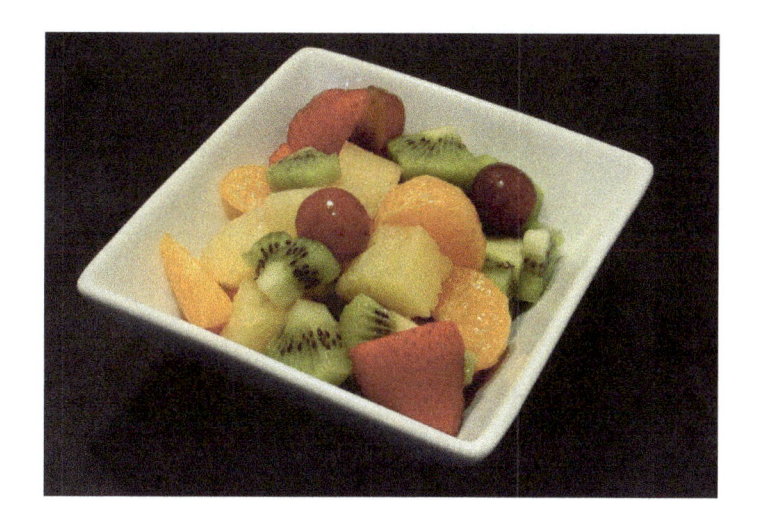

***Preparation Time**: 15 minutes*
***Servings**: 4*
Ingredients:

2 Kiwis, cubed
2 apples, cubed
1 cup grapes, halved
½ can sliced pineapples
1 cup blueberries
½ Tablespoon lime juice
Honey

Directions:

In a big bowl, mixed all the fruits together.

Add the lime juice.
Slowly add honey to suit your taste.
Refrigerate and serve chilled.

Almond Pancakes

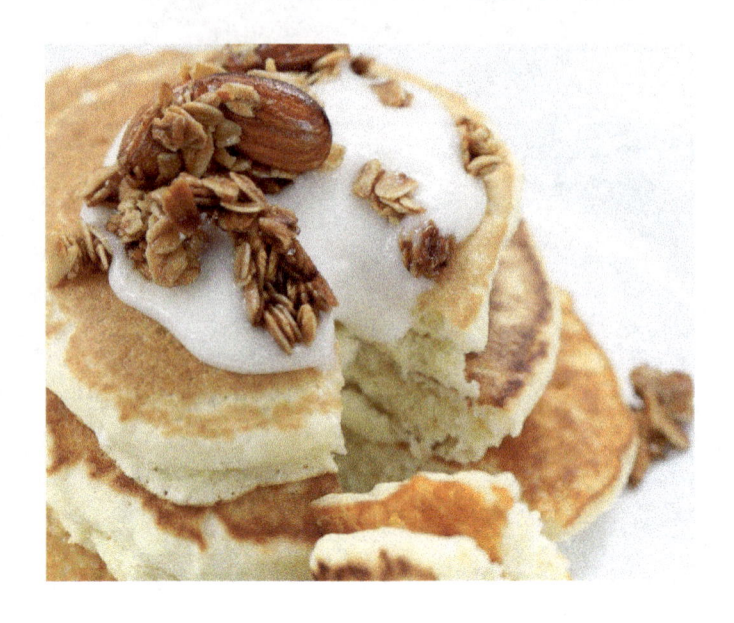

Cooking Time: 30 minutes
Servings: 2
Ingredients:

1 cup almond flour
½ cup applesauce (unsweetened)
2 large eggs
¼ cup water
¼ tsp coconut oil
fresh berries

Directions:

Mix together almond flour, applesauce, eggs, water and salt with a fork. When done, it should appear fluffier than ordinary pancake mix.

On a greased pan or skillet, drop about ¼ cup of the mixture.

When bubbles start to form, flip the pancake and cook for another 2 minutes.

You can add more coconut oil when necessary to prevent the mixture from sticking.

Serve with fresh berries on top.

Shrimp Omelette with Avocado

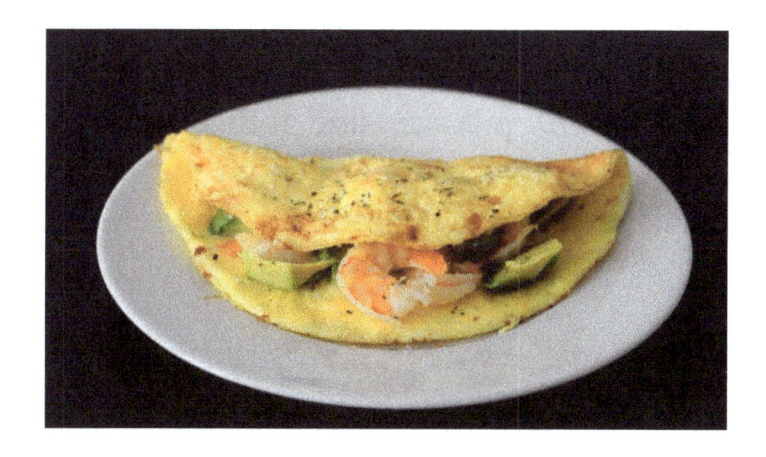

Cooking Time: 25 minutes
Servings: 2
Ingredients:

½ lb shrimp, peeled and de-veined
1 large tomato, diced
1 avocado, diced
1 tsp coconut oil
5 eggs

Directions:

Sautee shrimp until pink.
Mix the diced tomato and avocado; season with salt and pepper to taste.
In a small bowl, beat eggs chop cooked shrimps.

Heat skillet and add coconut oil. Pour half of the beaten eggs. Make sure the egg covers the entire skillet bottom.

When satisfied with firmness, place half of the chopped shrimps unto one side of the omelet. Fold another half of the omelet over the shrimps. Serve with tomato and avocado topping.

Almond Churros Waffles

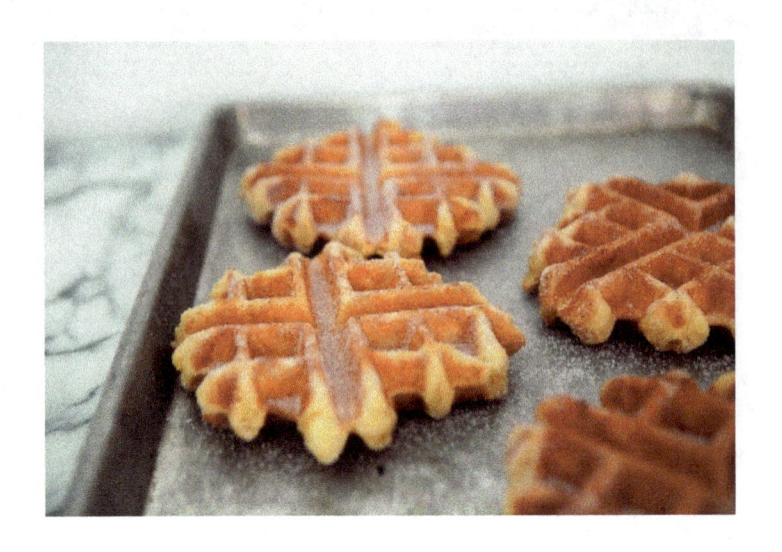

Cooking Time: 25 minutes
Servings: 2
Ingredients:

1.5 cups almond flour
½ tsp baking soda
⅓ cup coconut milk
2 eggs, beaten
1 tbsp honey
1 tsp vanilla extract
3 tbsps coconut oil
1/3 cup coconut sugar
A pinch of salt

Directions:

Thoroughly mix or blend together the almond flour, baking soda, and salt in a bowl.
Add coconut milk, eggs, honey, and vanilla extract and mix well.
Preheat waffle iron and place some of the mixtures in for cooking.
Place coconut oil in a wide-mouth bowl. Place the coconut sugar in a separate wide-mouth bowl.
After waffles are cooked, dip them into the melted butter first, making sure to soak them with oil, then place them into the coconut sugar to coat.
Serve them warm.

Vegetable with Hardboiled Eggs and Ham

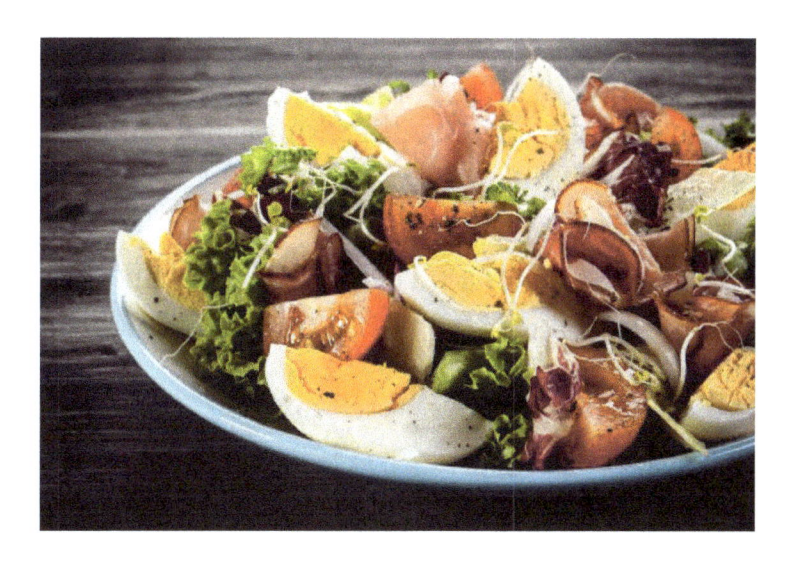

Cooking Time: 10 minutes
Servings: 2
Ingredients:

2 tbsps coconut oil
2 eggs
1 medium onion, sliced roughly
1 small carrot, sliced
1 large tomato, sliced
1-2 stalks of celery, chopped
1 small avocado, sliced
1 large broccoli, chopped

baby spinach, chopped roughly
8 slices of ham

Directions:

Boil water in a deep pot.
Gently drop eggs into boiling water and wait for six minutes before turning the stove off. Do not remove from boiling water.
Combine veggies on a large plate with ham.
Peel eggs and place one in the middle of the veggies
Add salt and pepper to taste.

Loaded Apricot Squares

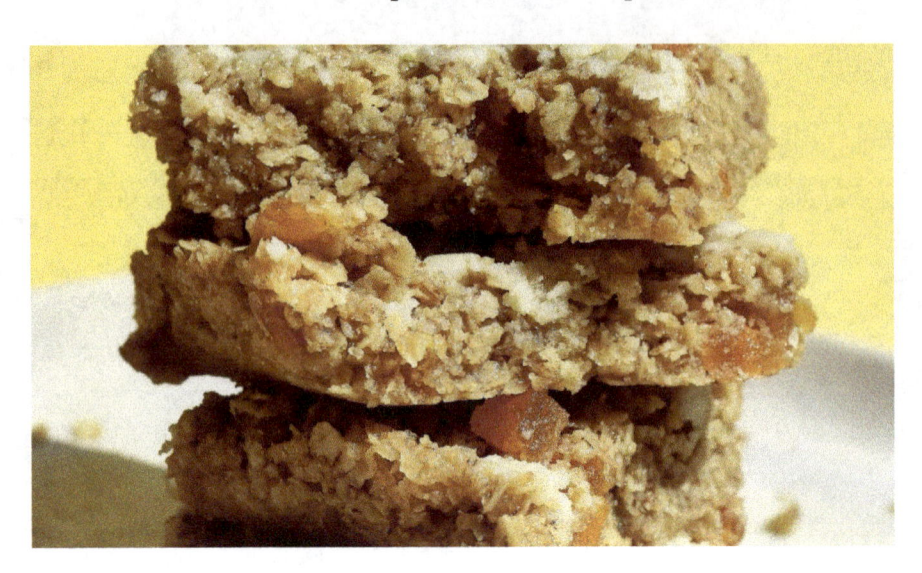

Cooking Time: 30 minutes
Servings: 6
Ingredients:

1 cup dried apricots
2 cups walnuts
2 organic eggs
¼ teaspoon sea salt
1 tablespoon vanilla extract

Directions:

Process walnuts and apricots in a mixer until well blended and coarse.

Add the eggs, salt, and vanilla and blend until the mixture forms a ball.

Spread the apricot mixture in a greased 9x9 inch baking dish.

Bake for 20 minutes at 350°. It is best to preheat the oven.

Serve when done baking and cool.

Breakfast Sausage with Mashed "Potato"

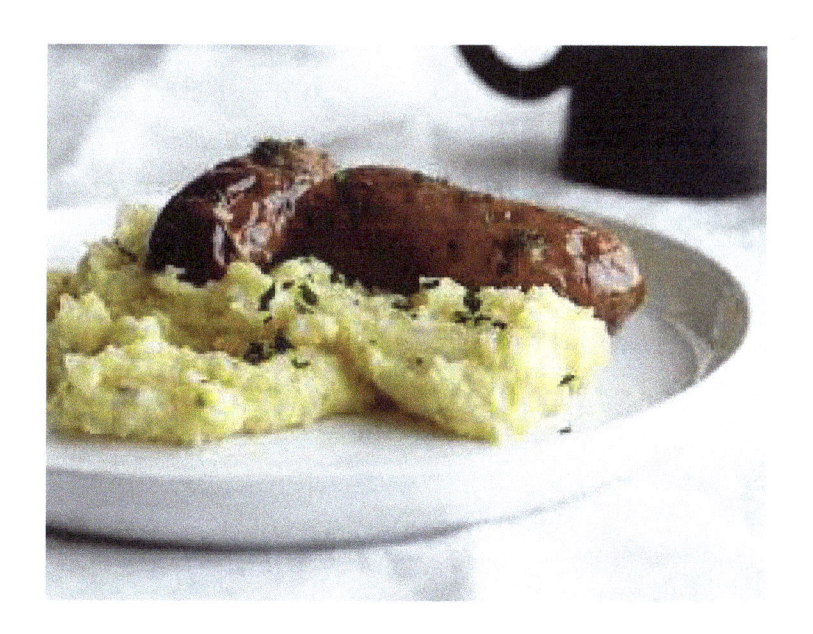

Cooking Time: 20 minutes
Servings: 2
Ingredients:

4 breakfast sausages
2 large cauliflowers
2 tbsps of grassfed butter
2 small cloves of garlic, sliced
Pinch of nutmeg
½ tsp. salt
More salt to taste

2 tbsps. coconut oil

Directions:

Heat some water in a steamer.
Wash and clean cauliflowers. Quarter them into manageable seizes for food processors.
When the steamer is ready, dump cauliflowers and garlic in and cook until tender.
Drain cauliflowers and garlic into coriander.
Put cauliflowers in the food processor; add the nutmeg and salt. Process until smooth.
You can store it in the refrigerator and reheat it when needed.
In a small pan, heat the coconut oil over medium heat.
Cook sausages until done.
Serve sausages with a side of mashed "potatoes".

Eggs Benedict

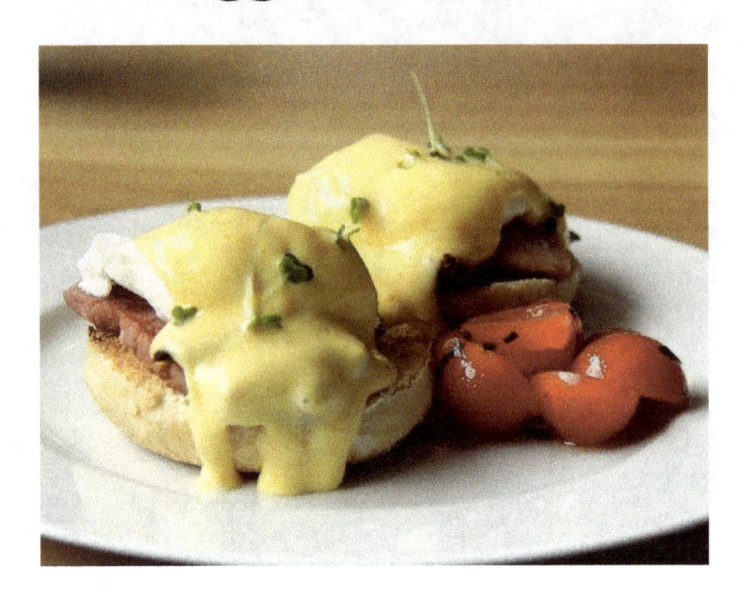

Cooking Time:10 minutes
Servings: 8
Ingredients:

8 eggs
8 strips of bacon
4 Paleo biscuits
Salt and pepper to taste

Directions:

Split Paleo biscuits in half. Toast all of them slightly.

Heat a skillet over medium high heat and place bacon in it.

Cook bacon until just slightly smoked or browned. Set aside.

Use bacon grease to cook eggs sunny side up style.

Arrange a bacon strip on top of muffin. Bacon can be cut or chopped.

Place a sunny side up egg on top of the bacon and sprinkle with salt and pepper to taste.

Stuffed Paleo Baguette

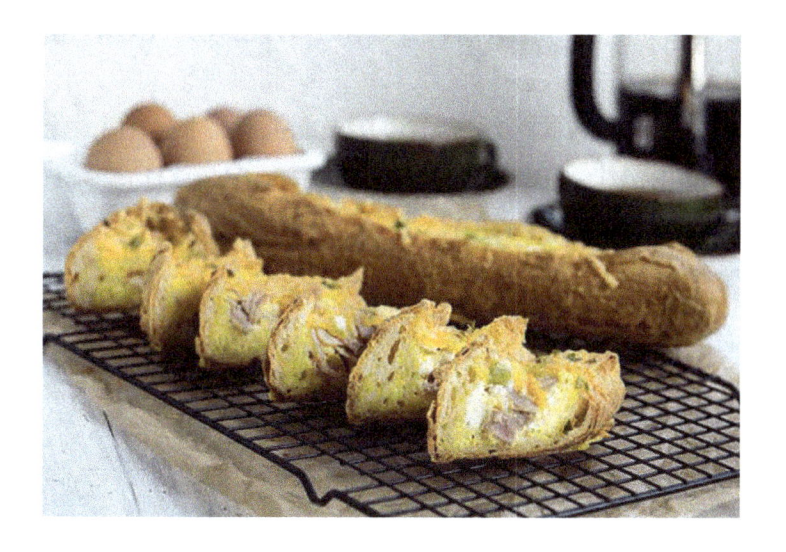

Cooking Time: 6-10 minutes
Servings: 4
Ingredients:

1 whole Paleo baguette
4 large eggs
3-4 spinach leaves, roughly chopped
1 large onion (white), diced

Directions:

Cut the baguette into smaller slices, about four parts. Make a deep hole in the middle of each.
You can also slice each part into half to make a sandwich.

Beat eggs in a medium-size bowl. Add the rest of the ingredients together with the egg.
Cook egg on a medium size pan over medium-high heat. Scramble.
Stuff the egg mixture into the holes of the baguette using a small spoon. Or if you sliced the parts into half, make a sandwich.
Serve warm.

Potato Pancakes

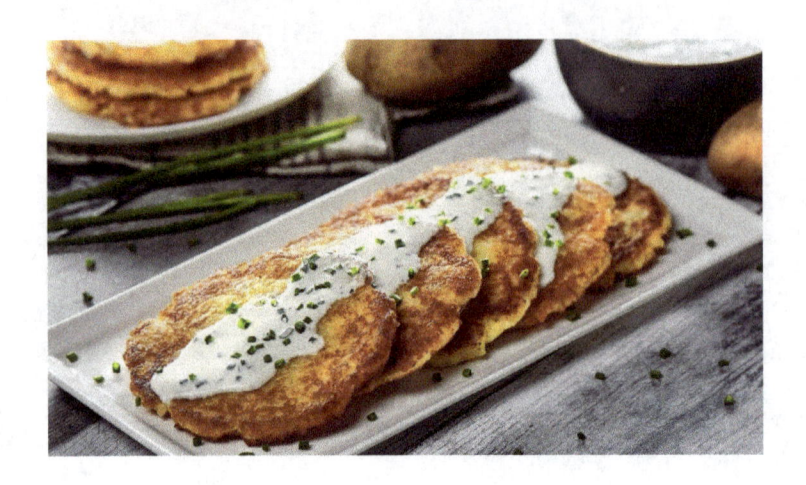

Cooking Time: 30 minutes
Servings: 4
Ingredients:

5 potatoes
3 eggs
3 tbsps. almond flour
1 onion
4 tbsps. coconut oil

Directions:

Peel potatoes and shred them.
Beat eggs in a large bowl. Add all the ingredients together, excluding coconut oil.
Heat the coconut oil in a pan in medium-high heat. Drop a spoonful of potato batter and flatten.

Each side should be cooked at around 4 minutes.

Ham and Eggs with Potato

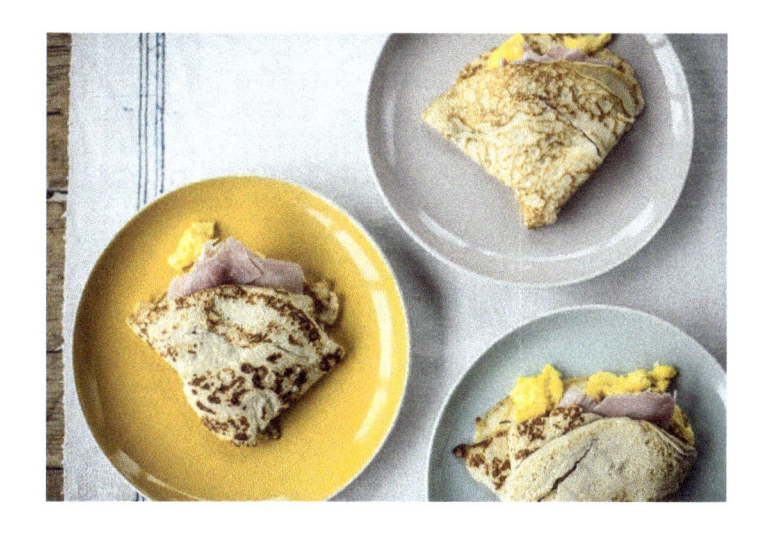

Cooking Time: 15 minutes
Servings: 2
Ingredients:

4 medium eggs
2 large potatoes cut into small wedges
3 slices of ham
Coconut oil for frying
Dill for garnish
Salt and pepper to taste

Directions:

Slice the ham into small slices, about two inches long. Set aside.

Deep fry potato wedges and when they are done, mix them with the sliced ham.

Cook eggs sunny side up.

Arrange potato and ham mix on two plates. Top with two sunny side-up eggs per plate.

Garnish with dill and sprinkle salt and pepper to taste.

Minced Pork on Fried Egg

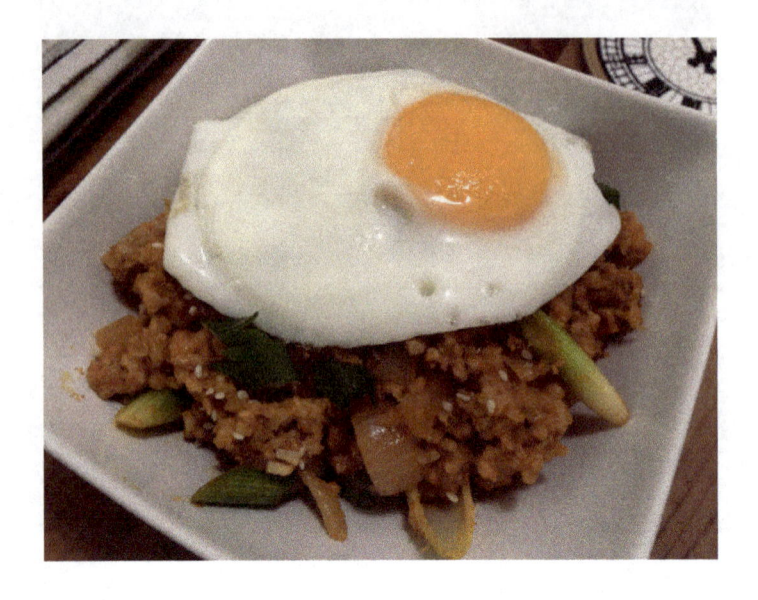

Cooking Time: 10 minutes
Servings: 1
Ingredients:

1 large egg
1 large tomato
1 spring onion leaf
¼ cup minced pork
2 tbsps coconut oil

Directions:

Brown minced pork in a pan over medium heat. Set aside.

Puree large tomato in a blender. Set aside.
Heat coconut oil in a small pan. Cook egg sunny side up; place in a plate when finished.
Place minced meat on the egg.
Pour some tomato puree over minced meat and egg.
Roughly chop the spring onion and use it as garnish.

Nutty French Toast

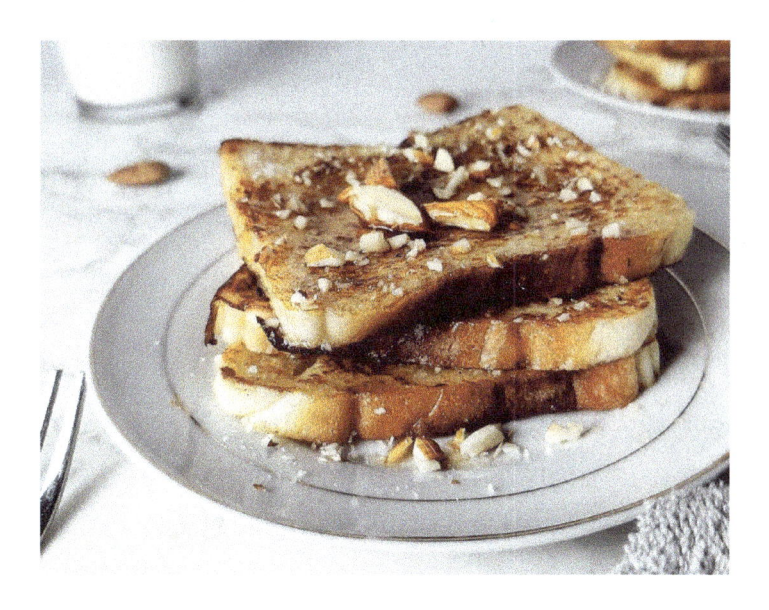

Cooking Time: 10 minutes
Servings: 1
Ingredients:

2 medium-sized slices of Paleo bread
2 medium eggs
½ cup chopped walnuts
1 tsp. cinnamon
1 tsp. nutmeg
½ cup Coconut oil

Directions:

Crack the eggs in a large bowl. Whisk well while adding the cinnamon and nutmeg.
Toast the bread lightly.
Soak lightly toasted bread into a large bowl with egg mixture.
While it is soaking, heat up the coconut oil in a shallow pan or skillet.
Cook the slices of bread until the egg mix browns.
Remove slice of bread from oil; sprinkle chopped walnuts and more cinnamon on the finished product.
You can also sprinkle some coconut sugar for sweetness.
Best served warm.

Raisin Bread with Cinnamon

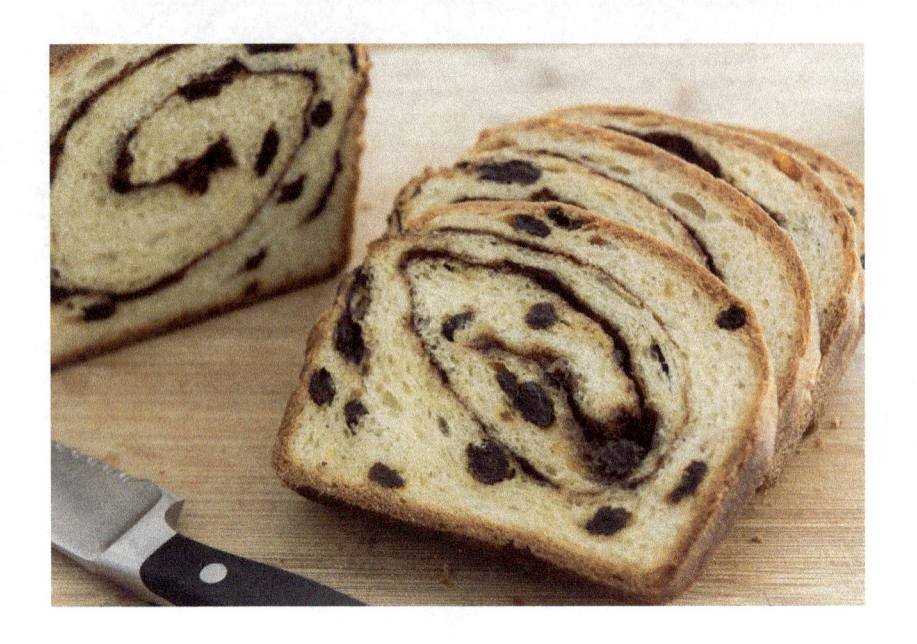

Cooking Time: 40 minutes
Servings: 10
Ingredients:

2 cups almond flour
2 tbsp. ground cinnamon
1 tsp. Baking soda
¼ tsp. sea salt
5 eggs
¼ cup honey
¼ cup coconut oil
2 tips. vanilla

½ cup raisins

Directions:

Preheat oven to 350 F.
Line a loaf pan with parchment paper.
Mix the almond flour with the baking soda, cinnamon, and salt in a bowl.
Combine with eggs, honey, melted coconut oil, and vanilla using an electric mixer.
Add dry ingredients to the wet ingredients and continue to mix.
Stir in the raisins when the mixture is ready to bake.
Put the batter into the lined baking dish.
Bread should be ready in 30 minutes or when a toothpick comes out clean.

Eggplant with Egg

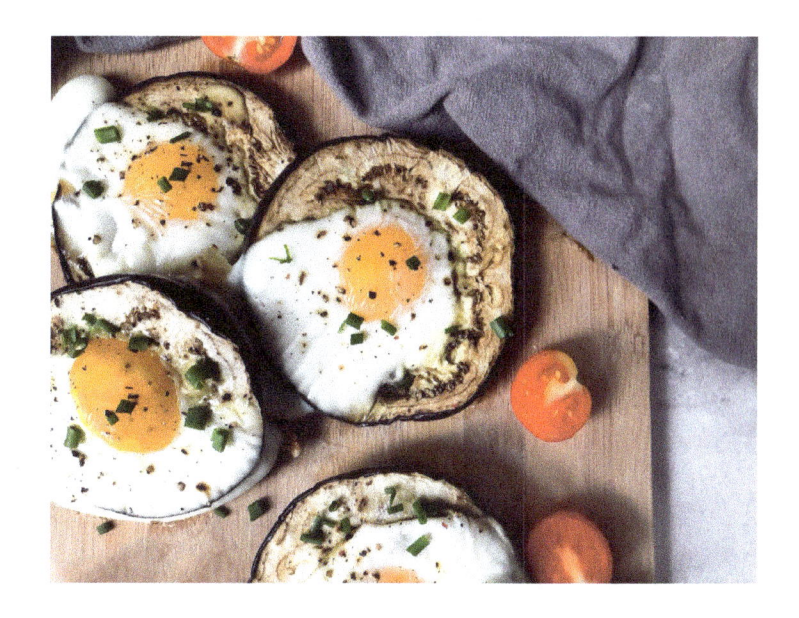

Cooking Time: 10 minutes
Servings: 3
Ingredients:

3 eggplant, sliced into discs
4 eggs
Coconut oil for frying
Salt and Pepper

Directions:

Preheat the skillet over medium-high heat. Pour a little coconut oil into the pan.

Beat the eggs well.
Dip each eggplant slice into the beaten eggs.
After dipping, immediately place the slices in the heated skillet for frying.
The eggplant slices can be fried together in the skillet.
They are ready when the eggs brown a little.
If there is any egg left over, make an omelet out of it and include it in the breakfast.
Add salt and pepper to taste.

Green-Eyed Smoothie

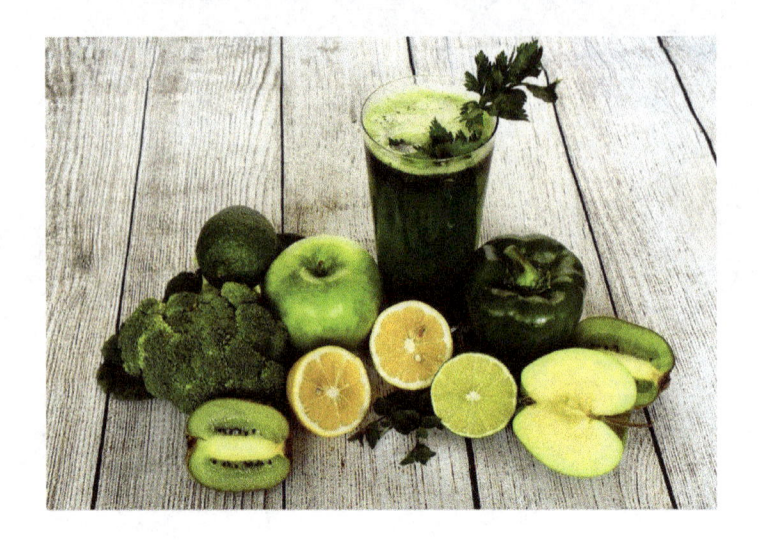

Cooking Time: 10 minutes
Serving: 2
Ingredients:

1 apple
1 pear
½ tsp. freshly grated ginger
2 Tbsp. sliced almonds
2 handfuls of spinach
1 small lemon
1 cup water

Directions:

Slice and quarter apple and pear while removing stems and seeds.
Pulse in a blender for a few seconds before adding the remaining ingredients.
Puree.

Chocolate Banana Pancake

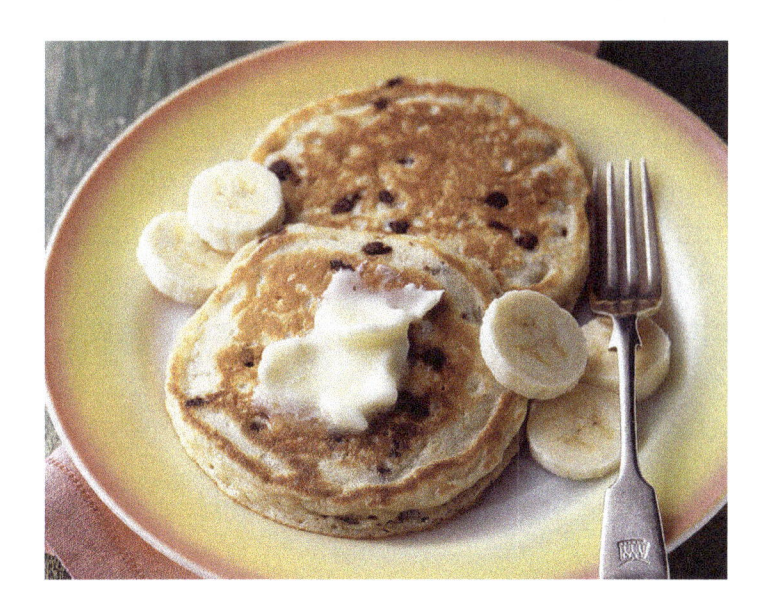

Cooking Time: 10 minutes
Servings: 6
Ingredients:

3 bananas, medium size
3 eggs
5 tablespoons full fat coconut milk
2 cup almond flour
¼ teaspoon baking soda
1 tablespoon coconut palm sugar
⅓ cup ground almonds
chocolate chips, about half a cup coconut oil for frying

Directions:

Mash the 3 bananas with a fork in a bowl and mix with the 3 eggs and coconut milk.
Mix the almond flour with the baking soda, salt and coconut sugar, ground almonds and chocolate chips in another bowl.
Combine the contents of both bowls in a larger bowl. Mix well.
Heat the coconut oil in the skillet and pour in about half a cup of batter.
Cook both sides well.

Breakfast Sausage Patty

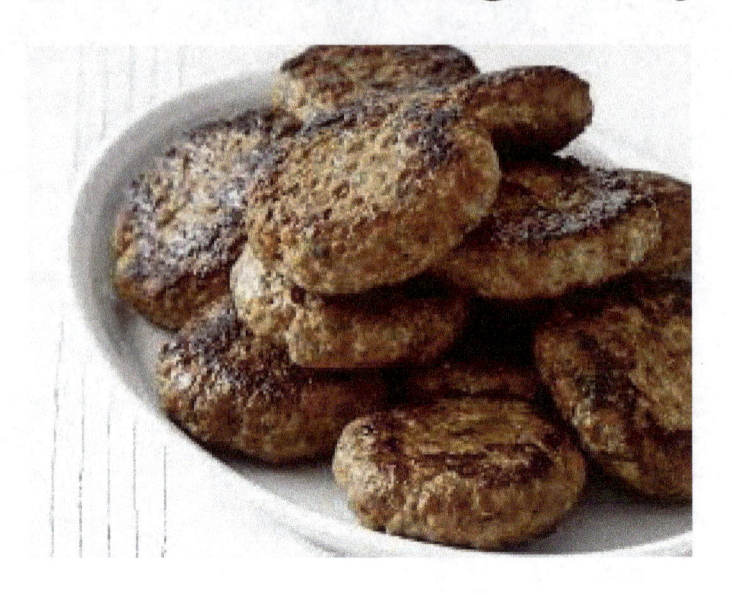

Cooking Time: 20 minutes
Servings: 10
Ingredients:

1 pound of ground pork
1 tsp. onion powder
¼ tsp. nutmeg
¼ tsp. cumin
¼ tsp. oregano
¼ tsp. black pepper
¼ tsp. red pepper flakes
¼ tsp. ground ginger
1 tsp. of salt

1 1/2 tsp poultry seasoning (or mix your own using 1/2 tsp each of sage, thyme, and basil)
1 egg, beaten

Directions:

Mix all of the ingredients together. Many people swear mixing by hand works very well.
After thoroughly mixing, put in a bowl and store in the refrigerator to allow flavors to blend.
After a few hours, remove from refrigerator and start forming patties.
Fry on medium high heat for about 3 minutes on one side, and then flip to cook the other side. The time needed to cook one side is dependent on how thick the patty is.

Paleo Granola

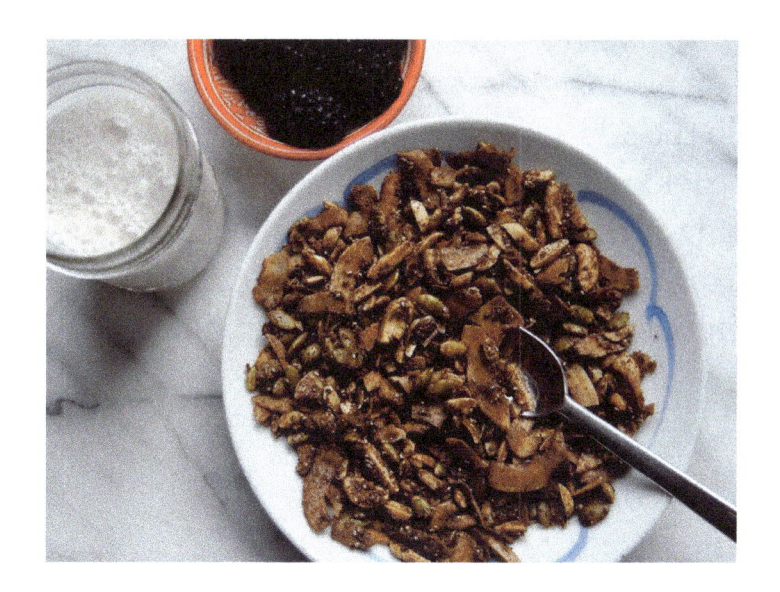

Cooking Time: 30 minutes
Servings: 6
Ingredients:

1/2 cup coconut oil
1.5 cups almond flour
1/4 cup of raw honey
2 tsp. ground cinnamon
2 tsp. vanilla extract
1 tsp. sea salt
1 cup raisins
1 cup other dried fruits of your choice

Directions:

Preheat your oven to 275F and mix the first six ingredients together.
Mix in the add-in ingredients of your choice.
Line cookie sheet with baking paper or parchment.
Spread the dough onto the lined sheet.
Bake for 10 minutes, then stir once or twice before continuing to bake for another 10 minutes.
Remove from oven and let it cool.

Beef Patties with Fennel

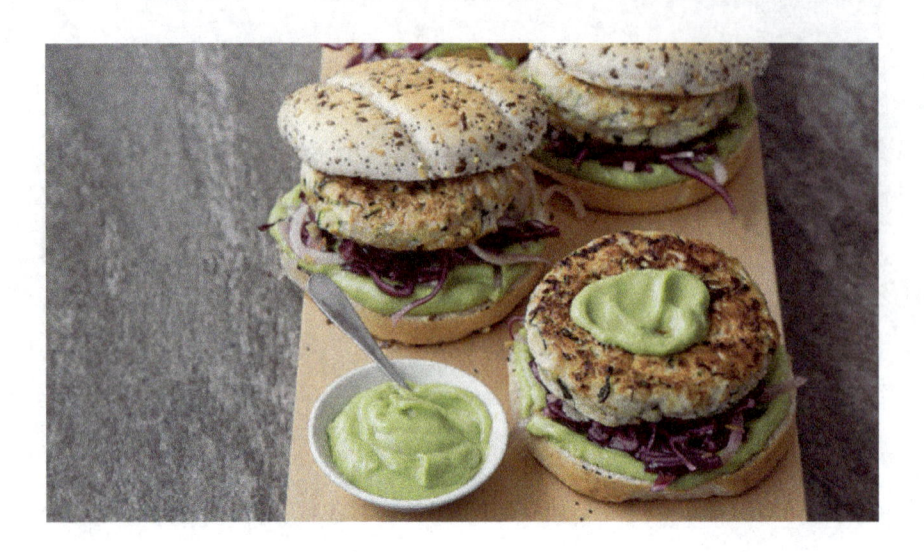

Cooking Time: 20 minutes
Servings: 4
Ingredients:

1 lb. ground beef
1 tsp. Fennel seed
¾ tsp. Anise seed
½ tsp. paprika
1-2 Tbsp. extra virgin coconut oil; for cooking

Directions:

Grind fennel seed and anise seed in a mortar and pestle or any other way.

In a large mixing bowl, mix the ground-up fennel and anise seeds with the ground beef.

Form the meat into patties, no more than an inch thick.

Heat the coconut oil to medium-high in a skillet. Cook the patties on one side for around ten minutes and flip it to cook for another eight minutes on the other side. Do not overcook!

Salmon Fillets with Almond Meal

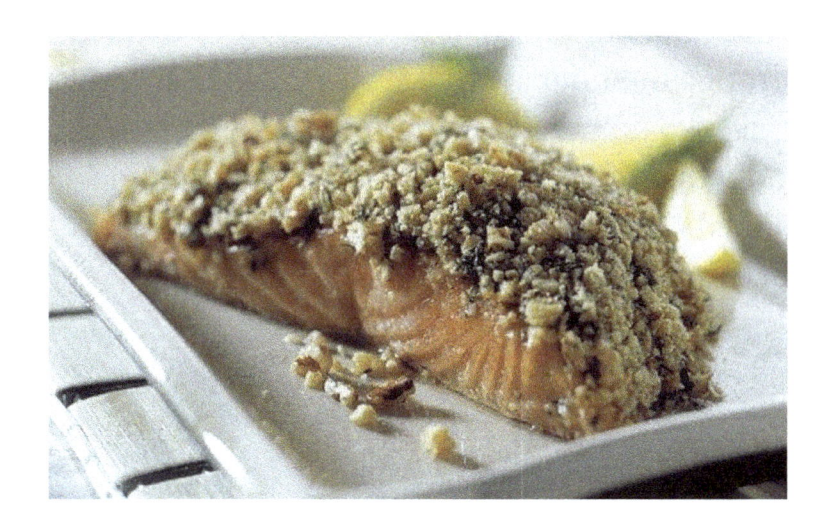

Cooking Time: 20 minutes
Servings: 4
Ingredients:

1 lb. salmon fillets with skin
¾ cup almond meal
½ tsp. ground coriander
½ tsp. ground cumin
1 large lemon
coconut oil

Directions:

The oven should be preheated to 360° F.

Mix the almond meal, coriander and cumin in a bowl.
Juice the lemon and shower the juice on the salmon fillets.
Lightly rub fillets with the almond meal mixture to coat both sides.
Arrange the fillets with the skin side down on a lightly greased baking tray.
Cook for 15 minutes, or try to flake a fillet to see if it is cooked.
Serve warm—season with salt and pepper.

Chicken in a Blanket

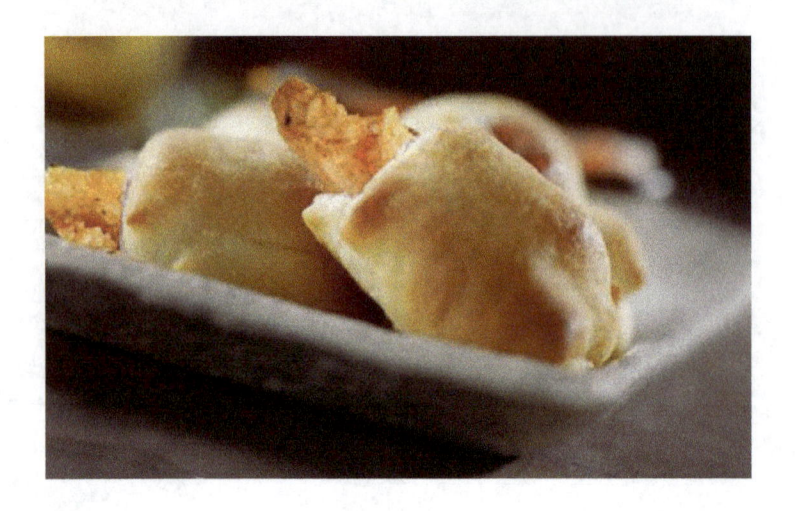

Cooking Time: 20 minutes
Servings: 4
Ingredients:

4 chicken thighs, better without skin
4 tbsp. fresh cilantro, finely chopped
long strips of bacon
Salt and pepper

Directions:

Lay the chicken thighs open on a clean surface
Add a dash of pepper and some cilantro on it.
Fold the chicken thighs close and wrap with the long strips of bacon.

Place the thighs on a baking tray or dish.
Bake for 20 minutes at 200 Celsius. It is best to preheat the oven.

Fruity Chicken

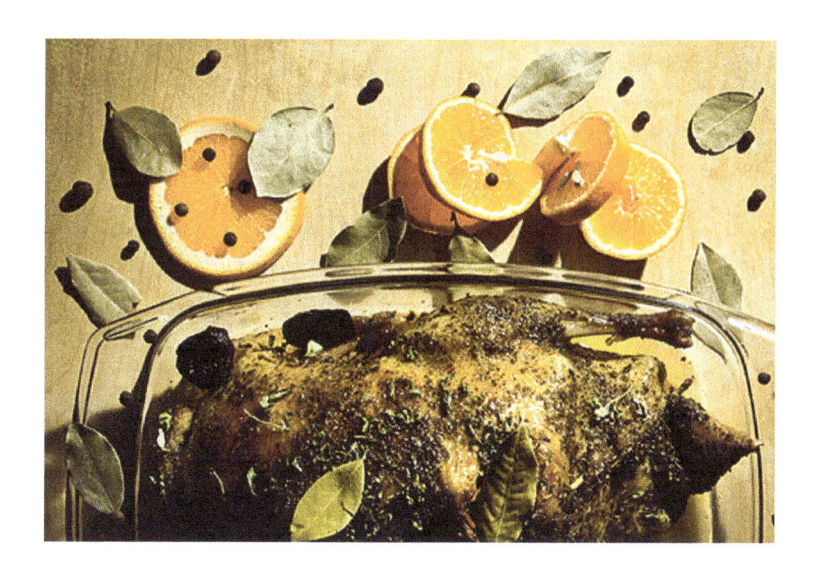

Cooking Time: 1.5 hour
Servings: 4
Ingredients:

8 large chicken thighs with skin
12 Tbsp. olive oil (divided)
2 medium white onions, diced
1 celery stalk, diced
2 small garlic cloves, minced
3 medium apples, cored
½ cup raisins
½ cup walnuts, chopped
2 eggs, beaten well
2 tsps. dried tarragon

Directions:

Preheat oven to 350.
Chop the onions, celery, garlic. Dice apples
Heat some olive oil in a skillet over medium-high heat.
Put the onions, celery, and garlic into the skillet.
Sauté until onion is translucent and celery is tender.
Remove from heat and add the apples, raisins, walnuts, and eggs. Set aside.
Pull the skin away from the chicken thighs without actually removing it.
Place the apple mix in the space between the skin and meat.
Line a baking dish with foil and place the chicken thighs on it. Skin facing up.
Mix the remaining olive oil in a small bowl with the tarragon. With a brush, baste the olive oil on the chicken. You may need to baste the chicken every fifteen to twenty minutes while baking.
Bake for about an hour without any covering.

Tuna in Mushroom Caps

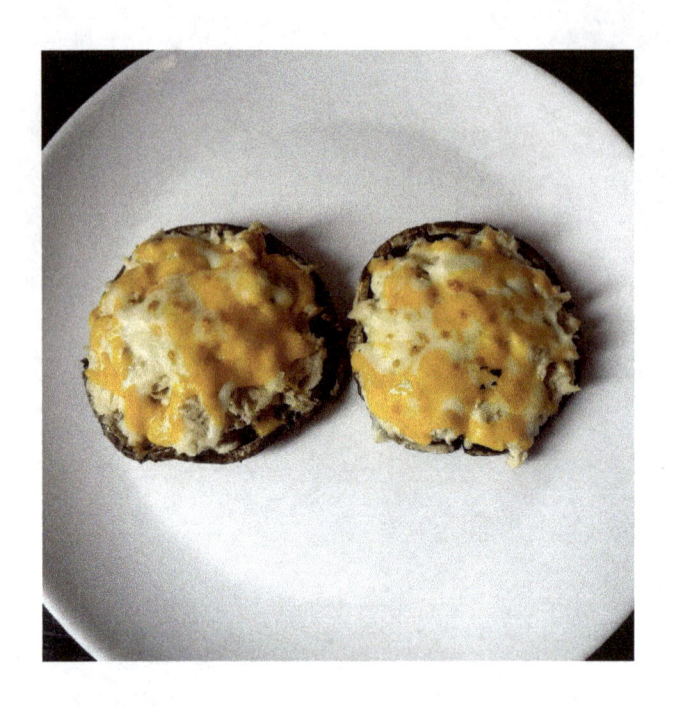

Cooking Time: 30 minutes
Servings: 4
Ingredients:

4 portobello mushroom caps
3 cans yellowfin tuna in oil, drained
½ tsp. garlic powder
½ tsp freshly ground black pepper
4 Tbsp. capers, rinsed
coconut oil to grease baking sheet
1 medium avocado

Directions:

Preheat oven to 450° F.
Mix tuna, garlic powder, black pepper, and capers together in a bowl.
Stuff the tuna mixture into the portobello caps. Arrange the portobello caps on a lightly greased baking tray and bake for 15-20 minutes.
You can also wait for the caps to turn brown and become somewhat tender, as a sign that they are cooked.
Slice open the avocado, remove the seed. Slice the meat into thin slices and add them to the portobello caps as garnish.
You can change the avocado into raisins or dill for a different taste.

Salmon and Caper Salad with Lemon

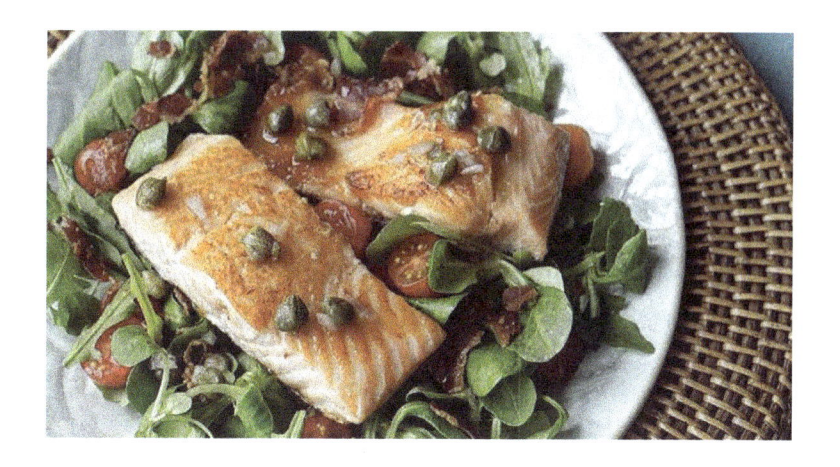

Cooking time: 10-15 minutes
Servings: 3
Ingredients:

1 pound flaked salmon
1 medium size lemon
2 tbsps. capers
1 tsp. dill (chopped)
1 stalk of celery (chopped)
Extra virgin olive oil for drizzling
Salt and pepper

Directions:

Clean lemon and get some zest before juicing it. Set aside. If you are using salmon fillets, season them with salt and pepper before baking them at 350 degrees in the oven for 10 minutes. Check if they are flaky for doneness.

Flake the salmon fillets; place flakes in a large bowl. Add lemon juice and zest into the salmon flakes and mix well.

Add capers, celery and dill. Mix well

Drizzle some extra virgin olive oil and season with salt and pepper.

Oyster Omelette

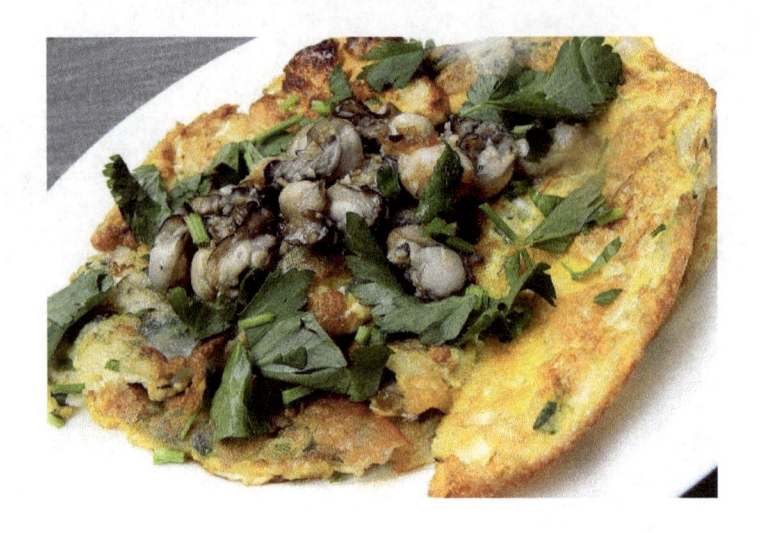

Cooking Time: 15 minutes
Servings: 3
Ingredients:

1 can oysters
2 medium eggs
2 tbsp. coconut oil
Pinch of ground black pepper

Directions:

Carefully open the jar of oysters, drain and set aside.
Heat the oil in a shallow skillet over medium heat.
Beat the eggs with a whisk.
Combine oysters with egg.

Pour the oysters and egg mixture into the heated skillet. Make sure the bottom of the pan is totally covered.

Fold the frittata over or flip it over to cook the other side.

Serve warm.

Sausage, Bacon and Egg Breakfast

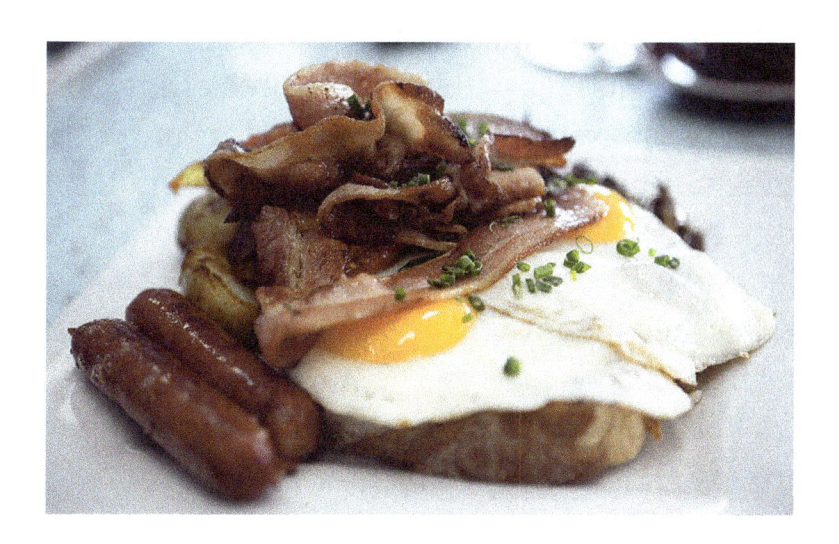

Cooking Time: 15 minutes
Servings: 2
Ingredients:

4 pcs sausages
6 strips bacon
4 medium eggs
1 cup cherry tomatoes
4 pcs olives
4 leaves lettuce
Coconut oil for frying
Water

Directions:

Preheat pan in medium heat, pour two tbsps. Of water into pan while heating.
Poke the sausages with a fork to break the skin
Place the sausages into the pan and cover.
Cook sausages for about ten to fifteen minutes or until some oil from the sausages come out.
Set aside.
In another shallow pan, place bacon on medium-high heat.
Cook bacon according to your preferences. (crispy or browned). Set aside bacon grease.
Quarter half a cup of cherry tomatoes.
Halve the olives.
Heat bacon grease and crack the eggs into the pan. Stir in the quartered cherry tomatoes and scramble the eggs.
On a big plate, spread two lettuce leaves. Place remaining cherry tomatoes and olives on the lettuce leaves. Arrange the bacon, sausages and eggs on the plate.

Potato and Mushroom Medley

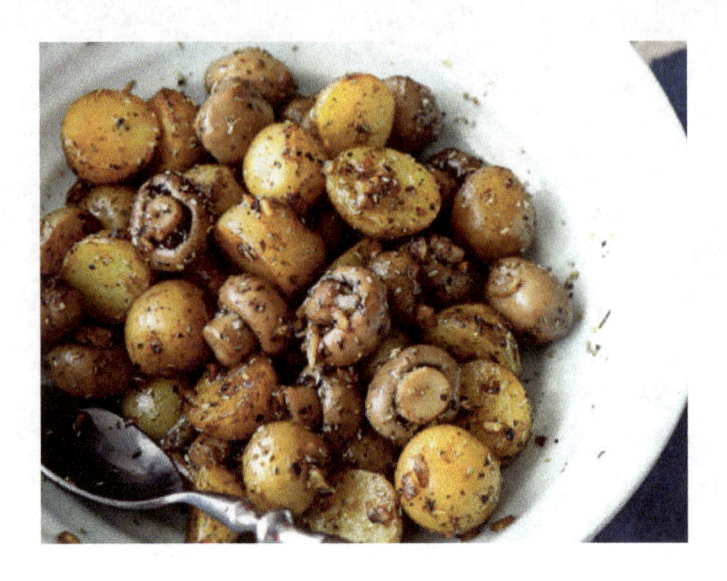

Cooking Time: 20 minutes
Servings: 2-3
Ingredients:

¼ lb. marble (or baby) potatoes, quartered or halved
½ cup champignons, halved
1 cup cherry tomatoes, halved
Salt and pepper to taste
Coconut oil

Directions:

Heat ½ cup coconut oil in a deep pot.

While waiting for the oil to heat up, add salt unto the quartered potatoes. Mix well.

When oil in pot is ready for deep frying, place the potatoes carefully into it.Potatoes should be done in seven-ten minutes. Set aside.

In a skillet over medium heat, transfer some of the oil used for deep frying.

Place all the mushrooms and cherry tomatoes in the skillet.

When tomatoes start wilting, mix in the fried potatoes and stir frequently.

Serve warm. Add salt and pepper to taste.

Dried Cherry-Sage Scoth Eggs

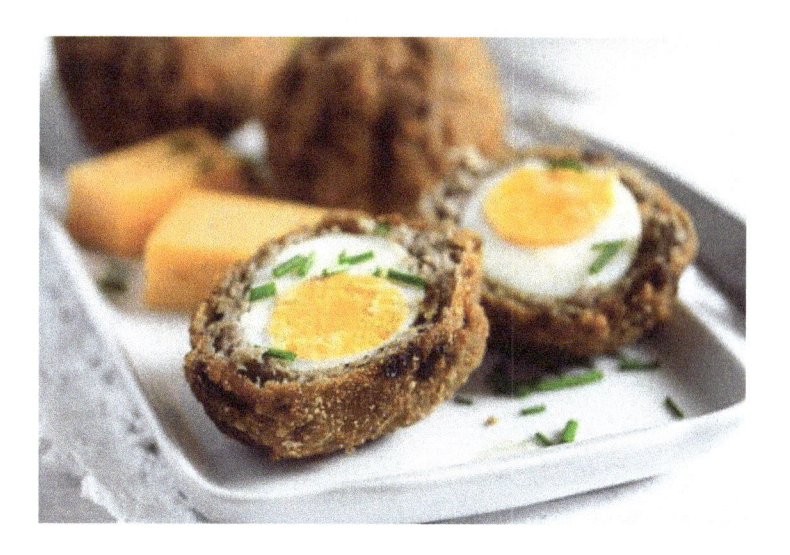

Cooking Time: 20 minutes
Servings: 2-3
Ingredients:

1 pound lean ground pork
½ cup snipped no-sugar-added dried cherries
2 tablespoons snipped fresh sage
1 tablespoon snipped fresh marjoram
1 teaspoon freshly ground black pepper
¼ teaspoon freshly ground nutmeg
⅛ teaspoon ground cloves
4 hard-cooked large eggs, cooled and peeled*
½ cup almond flour

1 teaspoon dried sage, crushed
½ teaspoon dried marjoram, crushed
2 tablespoons extra virgin olive oil
Dijon-Style Mustard

Directions:

Preheat oven to 380 F and coat a baking pan with parchment paper or foil; set aside. In a large bowl, combine pork, cherries, fresh sage, fresh marjoram, pepper, nutmeg, and cloves.
Shape pork mixture into four equal patties.
Place one egg on each patty.
Shape the patty around each egg. In a shallow pie plate, combine almond flour, dried sage, and dried marjoram.
Roll each sausage-coated egg in the almond flour mixture to coat.
Place on the prepared baking sheet.
Drizzle with olive oil.
Bake for about 30 min or until sausage is cooked through and serve with Dijon-style Mustard.

Eggs Shakshuka

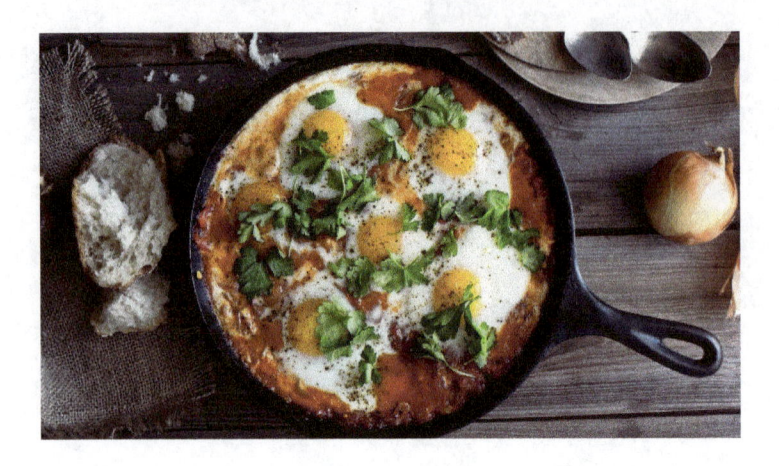

Cooking Time: 35 minutes
Servings: 2-3
Ingredients:

¼ cup extra virgin olive oil
1 large onion, halved and thinly sliced
1 large red sweet pepper, thinly sliced
1 large orange sweet pepper, thinly sliced
1 teaspoon ground cumin
½ teaspoon smoked paprika
½ teaspoon crushed red pepper
4 cloves garlic, minced
2 jars of roasted organic tomatoes without salt
6 eggs
Black pepper
¼ cup snipped fresh cilantro
¼ cup shredded fresh basil

Directions:

Preheat the oven to 380°F then in a large ovenproof skillet, heat oil over medium.
Add onion and sweet peppers and cook and stir for 5 minutes or until vegetables are tender.
Put cumin, paprika, crushed red pepper, and garlic; cook and stir for 2 minutes.
Stir in tomatoes, then bring to boiling; reduce heat.
Simmer without a lid for about 10/12 minutes or until thickened.
Crack eggs into skillet over tomato mixture.
Transfer the skillet to the preheated oven.
Cook without lid for about 7 minutes or until eggs are just cooked through and yolks are still soft.
Sprinkle with black pepper.
Garnish with cilantro and basil; serve immediately.

Trout with Shoestring sweet Potatoes

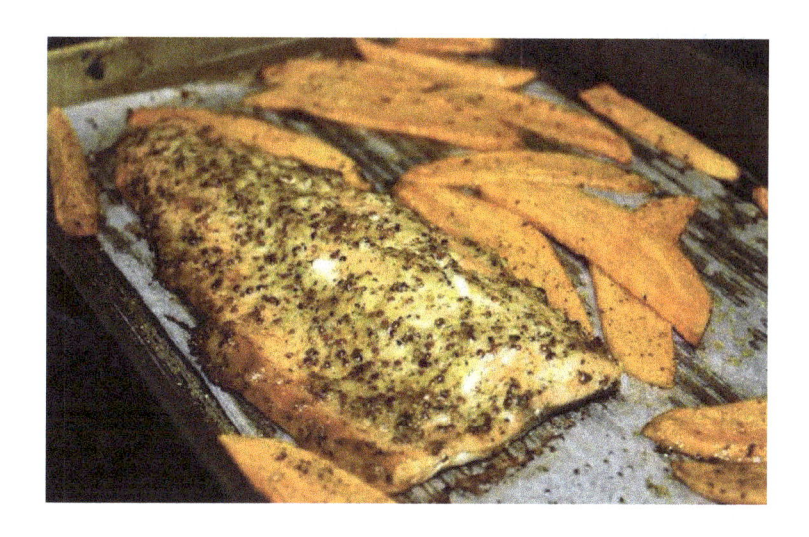

***Cooking Time:** 35 minutes*
***Servings:** 2-3*
Ingredients:

4 6-ounce fresh or frozen skinless trout fillets, ¼ to ½ inch thick
1½ teaspoons Smoky Seasoning
¼ to ½ teaspoon black pepper
3 tablespoons refined coconut oil
1½ pounds white or yellow sweet potatoes, peeled
Refined coconut oil for frying*
Chopped fresh parsley
Sliced scallions

Directions:

Preheat oven to 400°F. Thaw fish, if frozen.
Rinse fish; pat dry with paper towels.
Sprinkle fillets with Smoky Seasoning and, if desired, pepper.
In an extra-large oven going skillet heat 2 tablespoons of the oil over medium-high heat. Place fillets in skillet and bake, uncovered, for 6 to 8 minutes or until fish begins to flake when tested with a fork. Remove from oven.
Meanwhile, using a julienne peeler or mandoline fitted with the julienne cutter, cut sweet potatoes lengthwise into long thin strips.
Wrap potato strips in a double thickness of paper towels and absorb any excess water. In a large stockpot with at least 8-inch-tall sides, heat 2 to 3 inches of refined coconut oil to 365°F.
Carefully add potatoes, about one-fourth at a time, to the hot oil. Fry about 1 to 3 minutes per batch or until just starting to brown, stirring once or twice.
Quickly remove potatoes using a long slotted spoon and drain on paper towels.
(Potatoes can overcook quickly, so check early and often.) Be sure to heat oil back up to 365°F before adding each batch of potatoes.
Sprinkle trout with parsley and scallions; serve with sweet potato shoestrings.

Date Shakes

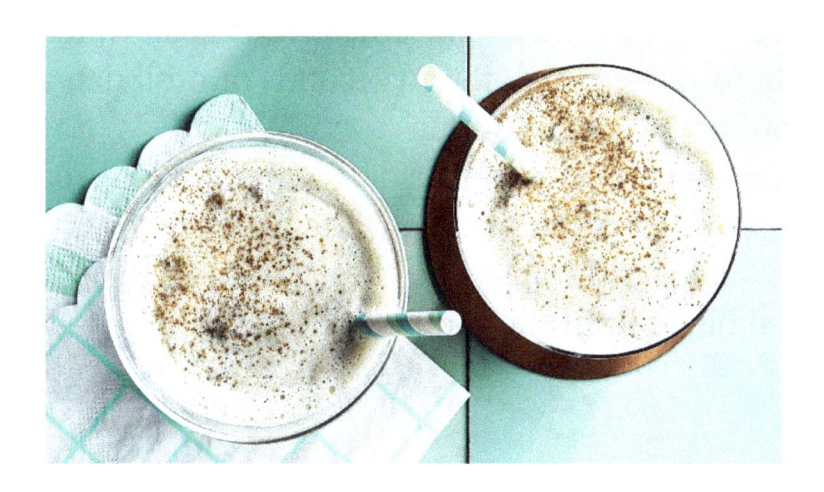

Cooking Time: 35 minutes
Servings: 2-3
Ingredients:

⅓ cup chopped, pitted Medjool dates
1 cup unsweetened almond or coconut milk
1 ripe banana, frozen and sliced
2 tablespoons almond butter
1 tablespoon egg white powder
1 tablespoon unsweetened cocoa powder
½ teaspoon fresh lemon juice
⅛ to ¼ teaspoon ground nutmeg

Directions:

In a small bowl combine dates and ½ cup water. Microwave on high for 30 seconds or until dates are softened; drain off water.
In a blender combine the dates, almond milk, banana slices, almond butter, egg white powder, cocoa powder (if using), lemon juice, and nutmeg. Cover and blend until smooth.

Apple-Flack Jacks

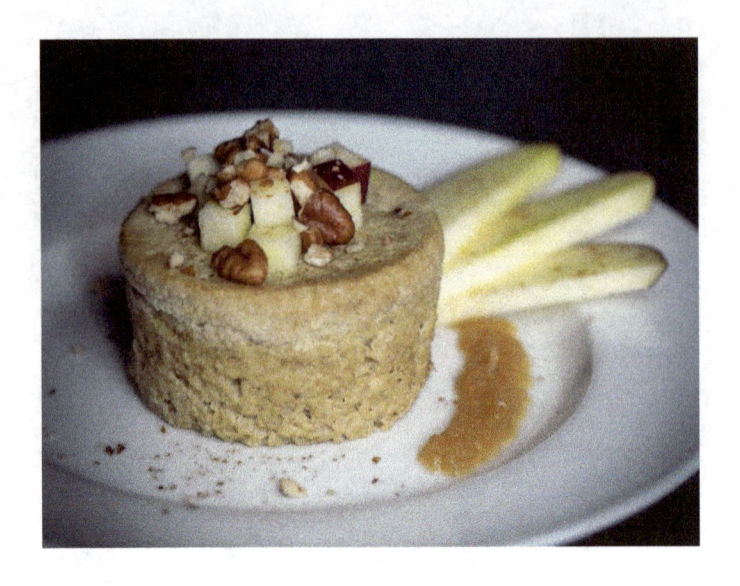

Cooking Time: 30 minutes
Servings: 2
Ingredients:

4 large eggs, lightly beaten
2 large unpeeled apples, cored and finely shredded
½ cup flax meal
¼ cup finely chopped walnuts or pecans
2 teaspoons finely shredded orange peel
1 teaspoon pure vanilla extract
1 teaspoon ground cardamom or cinnamon
3 tablespoons unrefined coconut oil

½ cup almond butter
2 teaspoons finely shredded orange peel
¼ teaspoon ground cardamom or cinnamon

Directions:

In a large mixing plastic bowl combine the eggs, chopped apple flax meal, nuts, orange peel, vanilla, and 1 teaspoon cardamom.
Stir until well combined.
Let the batter rest to thicken for about 7/10 minutes.
On a griddle or skillet, melt 1 tablespoon of the coconut oil over medium heat.
For each Apple-Flax Jack, drop about ⅓ cup batter onto the griddle, spreading slightly.
Cook over medium heat for 5 minutes on each side or until jacks are golden brown.
Meanwhile, in a small microwave-safe bowl, heat almond butter on low until spreadable.
Serve on top of Apple-Flax Jacks and sprinkle with orange peel and additional cardamom.

Rasperry Banana Sorbet

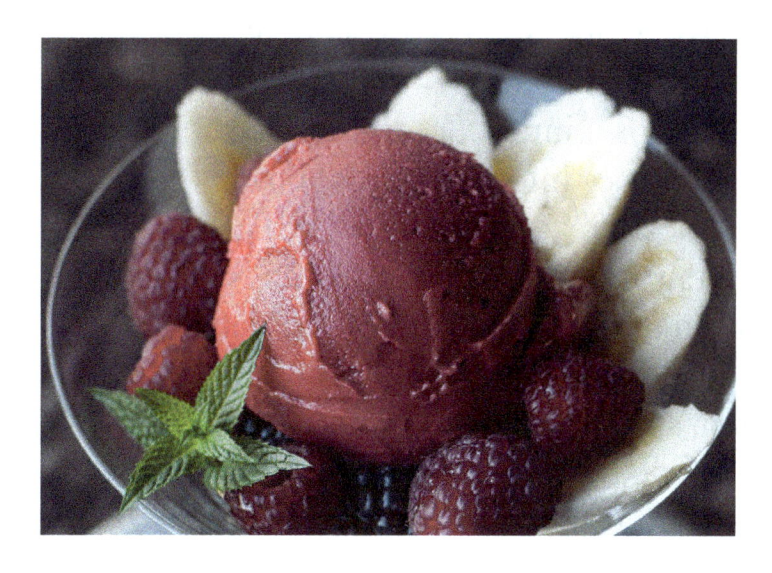

Cooking Time: 15 minutes
Servings: 2
Ingredients:

1 medium banana, cut into ½-inch slices
¾ cup fresh orange juice
2½ cups frozen unsweetened raspberries
Grated unsweetened chocolate (such as Scharffen Berger 99% cacao bar), toasted unsweetened coconut chips, and/or toasted slivered almonds

Directions:

Place banana on a small baking pan lined with waxed paper.

Cover loosely with another sheet of waxed paper.
Freeze for 2/3 hours or until completely firm.
Meanwhile, in a small saucepan, bring orange juice to boiling.
Boil for 6/8 minutes or until reduced to ⅓ cup.
Pour the juice into a heatproof bowl.
Chill for 30 to 50 minutes or until cold.
A food processor combines frozen banana slices, reduced orange juice, and frozen raspberries.
Cover and process until well combined but still frozen, stopping to stir often.
Sorbet will be very thick.
Immediately spoon into chilled serving bowls.
Serve immediately. (Or place the filled bowls in the freezer until serving time; let stand at room temperature for 5 minutes before topping and serving.) Sprinkle sorbet with chocolate, coconut chips, and/or almonds just before serving.

Fresh Fruit 'n Spinach Smoothie

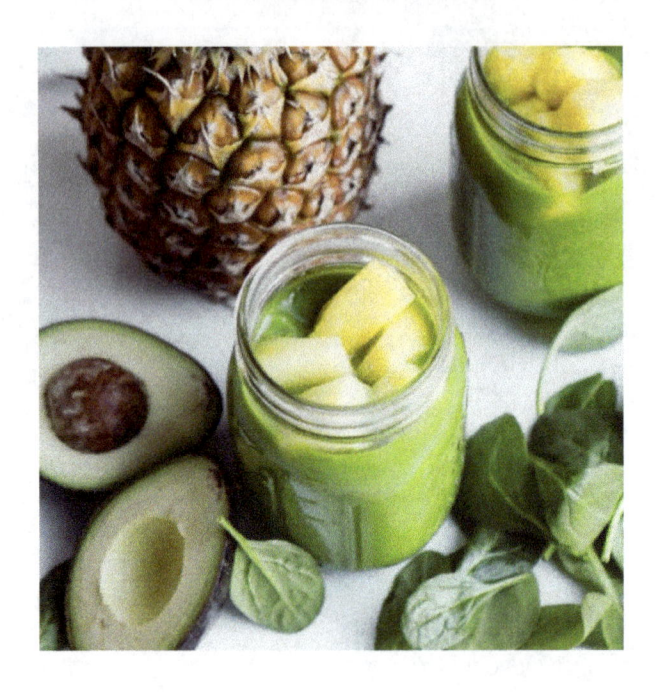

Cooking Time: 8 minutes
Servings: 2
Ingredients:

1/2 cup pure coconut milk
3/4 cup almond cream
1 fresh cold banana, peeled and chopped
1/4 cup flax seed
1 teaspoon raw honey
1/2 cup frozen strawberries

1/2 cup frozen raspberries
1 cup spinach leaves

Directions:

Put all the ingredients in a mixer and blend until smooth.
Chill, pour into glasses and serve.

Honey Glazed Pumpkin Donuts

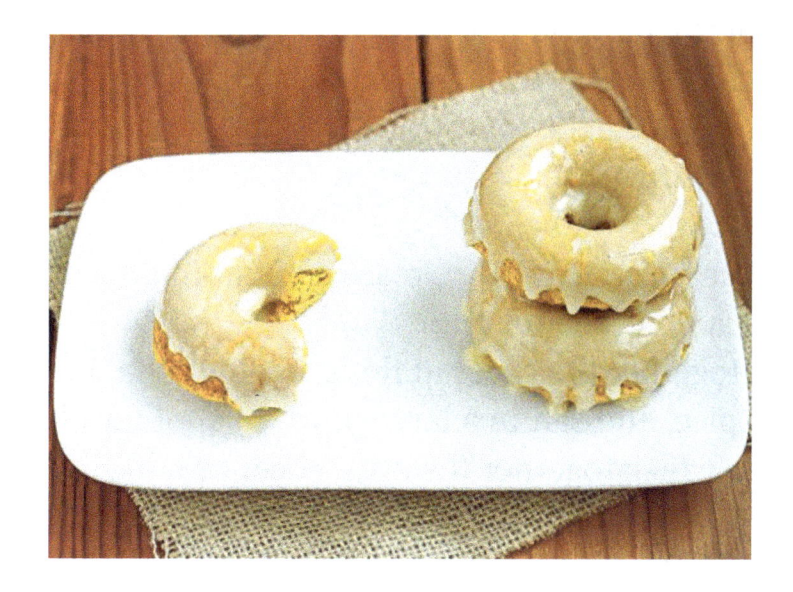

Cooking Time: 18 minutes
Servings: 2
Ingredients:

1/2 cup coconut flour
1/2 teaspoon baking soda
1 tablespoon pumpkin pie spice
1/4 teaspoon unrefined sea salt
2 pasture-fed, free-range eggs
1/2 cup pure light coconut milk
1/3 cup pumpkin puree
3 tablespoon pure maple syrup
2 tablespoon coconut oil + 1 tablespoon for greasing
Honey Glaze:

2 teaspoons coconut oil, softened
1 teaspoon raw honey, softened
1 tablespoon ground cinnamon
1/2 teaspoon pure vanilla extract

Directions:

Preheat oven to 350F. Grease a donut mold with 1 tablespoon coconut oil.
Mix together the coconut flour, baking soda, pumpkin pie spice, and salt in a large bowl. In another plastic bowl, whisk together the eggs, coconut milk, pumpkin, maple syrup, and coconut oil.
Add wet mixture to the dry mixture. Add a tablespoon of coconut milk if the batter is dry. Pour the batter into the donut mold.
Bake for 18 to 20 minutes, until donuts are golden brown or toothpick inserted in the center of donut comes out clean or with only a few crumbs sticking to it.
Cool donuts for 5 minutes in the pan then place in a wire rack.
Stir together all the ingredients for the glaze in a medium bowl. Set the bowl over hot water for 30 seconds; whisk mixture until creamy. Spread the glaze over the top of donuts using a butter knife.

Smoked Salmon Frittata

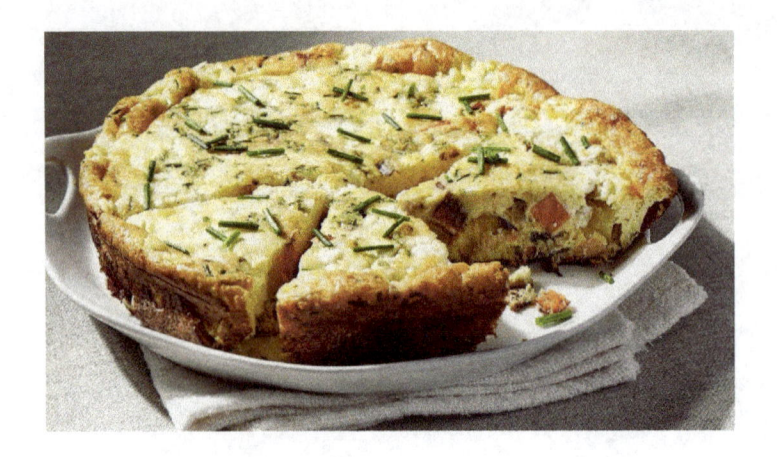

Cooking Time: 18 minutes
Servings: 2
Ingredients:

4 tablespoons olive oil
1/2 teaspoon of garlic
2 medium shallots, chopped
1/2 teaspoon unrefined sea salt
1/4 teaspoon ground black pepper
4 ounces pepper smoked salmon
4 red bell peppers, seeded and chopped
6 pasture-fed, free-range eggs
2 tablespoons pure coconut milk
1/4 teaspoon dried thyme
1/2 teaspoon dried rosemary
1 teaspoon fresh dill, chopped

Directions:

Preheat the oven to 350F.

Heat olive oil in a medium oven-safe skillet over medium heat.

Sauté garlic in olive oil until lightly browned. Stir in shallots, and season
with salt and pepper; cook, until shallots are translucent.

Add the salmon and red bell pepper, cook for about 5 minutes; stirring often.

Whisk together the eggs and coconut milk, stir in thyme, rosemary, and dill then pour mixture over the salmon in the skillet. Cook until the edges are firm.

Place the skillet in oven, and bake for 20 minutes, until golden brown.

Place frittata on a plate, cut into wedges, and serve.

Vanilla Berry Crepes

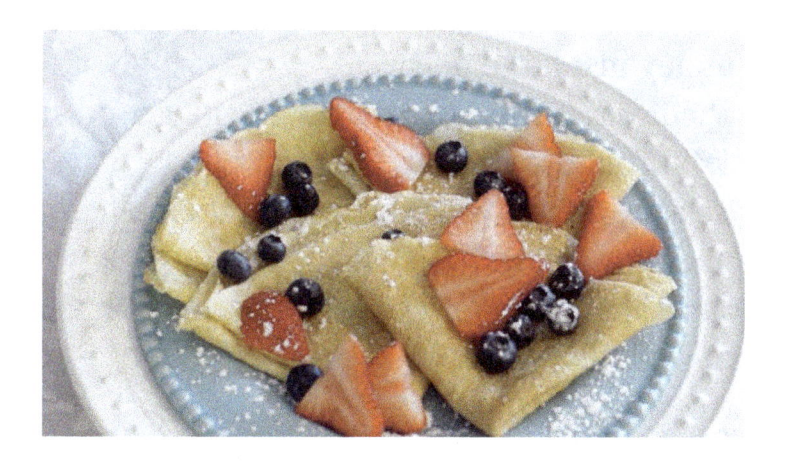

Cooking Time: 20 minutes
Servings: 2
Ingredients:

3 pasture-fed, free-range egg yolks
2 tablespoons pure vanilla extract
1 1/2 cups pure coconut milk
2 tablespoons raw honey
1 1/2 cups gluten-free almond flour
1/3 cup grass-fed raw milk butter, melted
1/4 teaspoon ground cinnamon
1/4 teaspoon nutmeg
1/2 teaspoon unrefined sea salt
Coconut oil for greasing
2 cups fresh strawberries, sliced
2 cups fresh blueberries

Directions:

Whisk together the egg yolks, vanilla, coconut milk, and honey in a large bowl.
Add the flour, butter, cinnamon, nutmeg, and salt; whisk thoroughly.
Grease a crepe pan with coconut oil then place pan over medium heat.
Pour and spread about 1/4 cup of batter (for each crepe) into the pan.
Brown crepes on both sides.
Fill crepes with strawberries and blueberries to serve.

Choco Banana Muffins

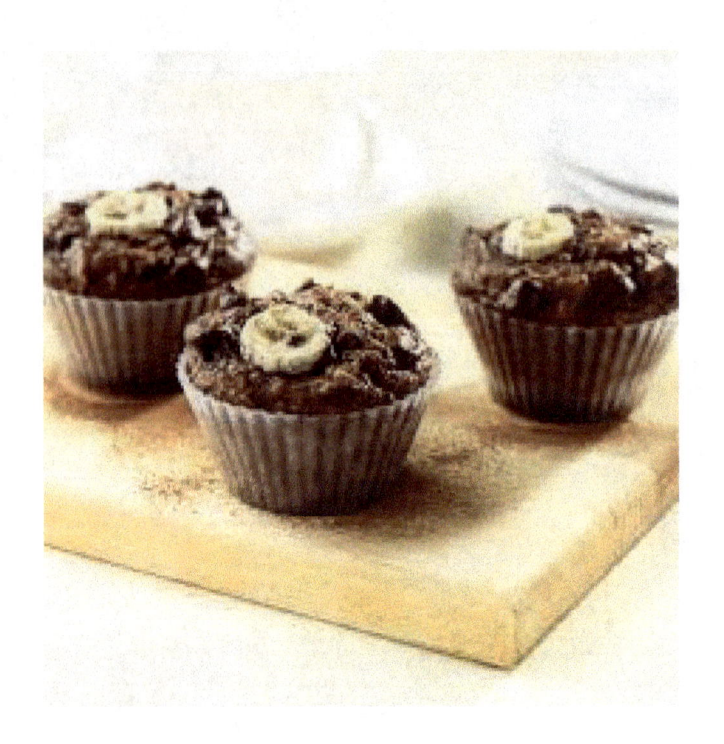

Cooking Time: 15 minutes
Servings: 2
Ingredients:

1/4 cup extra-virgin coconut oil, melted
1/2 cup raw honey
1/4 cup packed unrefined brown sugar
2 pasture-fed, free-range eggs
3 teaspoons pure vanilla extract
1 1/2 cups ripe bananas, mashed
1 3/4 cups almond flour

3 teaspoons baking soda
1 tablespoon cinnamon
1 cup walnuts, chopped
1/2 cup chocolate chips (70%-90% cocoa)

Directions:

Preheat oven to 350 degrees f. Line an 8-cup muffin pan with paper liners.
Whisk together coconut oil, honey, and brown sugar in a bowl.
Beat eggs in another bowl then stir in vanilla and mashed bananas. Mix together flour and baking soda then add to the egg mixture.
Stir in cinnamon, walnuts, and chocolate chips. Fill muffin cups half full.
Bake for about 15 minutes.

Turkey Veggie Meatza

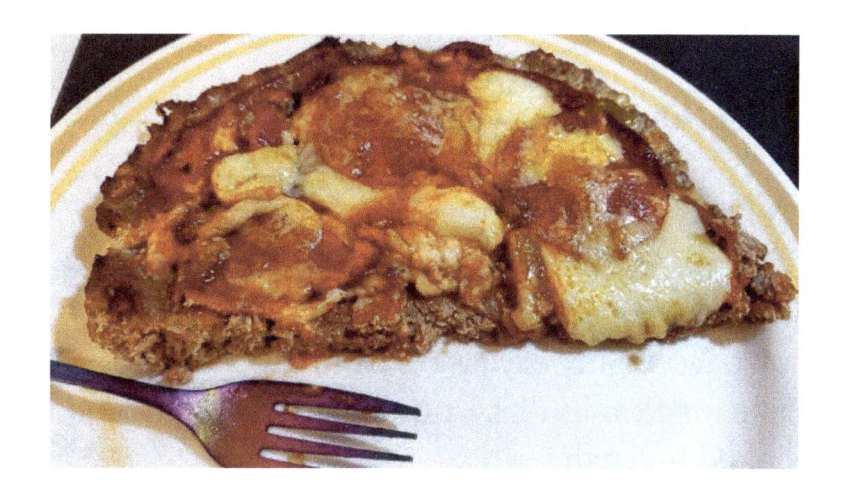

Cooking Time: 15 minutes
Servings: 2
Ingredients:

Olive oil for greasing
1 pound ground turkey
4 cloves garlic, crushed and chopped
1 tablespoon dried thyme
1 tablespoon dried basil
1/4 cup pure coconut milk
4 pasture-fed, free-range eggs
1/2 teaspoon garlic powder
1/2 teaspoon unrefined sea salt
1/2 teaspoon ground black pepper

1/2 cup zucchini, sliced
1/2 cup kalamata olives, chopped
1 1/2 cup mushrooms, sliced
1/2 cup roasted red peppers, chopped

Directions:

Preheat oven to 375 degrees f.
Grease a 7x7 inch baking dish with olive oil.
Mix together turkey, garlic, thyme, and basil in a bowl. Drain any excess oil from the meat.
Bake for 18 minutes, or until meat is just about cooked through.
Whisk together coconut milk, eggs, garlic powder, salt, and pepper in a bowl.
Stir in zucchini, kalamata olives, mushrooms, and roasted peppers.
Spread the egg mixture on top of the meat crust—return the dish into the oven.
Bake for 25-35 minutes, or until set. Cool then serve.

Carrot Walnuts Soufflé

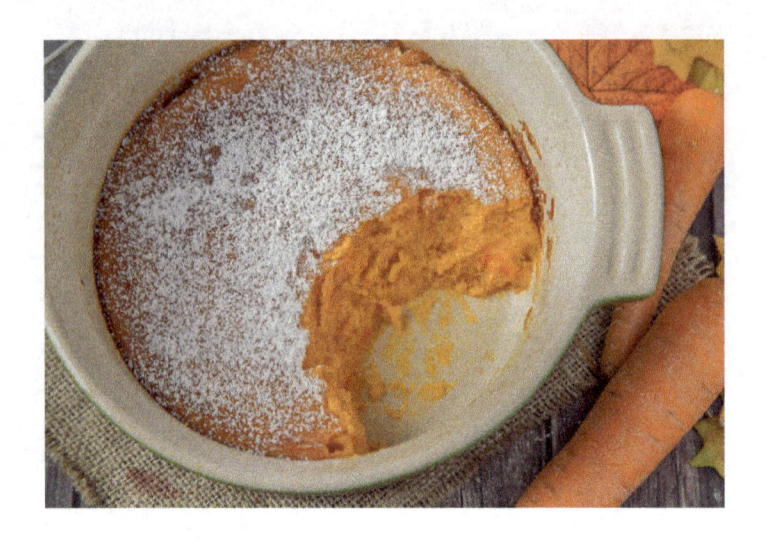

Cooking Time: 25 minutes
Servings: 2
Ingredients:

1 pounds carrots, chopped
1/3 cup organic coconut butter, melted
1/2 cup raw honey
3 tablespoons almond flour
1/4 teaspoon baking soda
1 1/2 teaspoon lemon juice
1 teaspoon pure vanilla extract
3 pasture-fed, free-range eggs, beaten
1 teaspoon ground cinnamon
1 teaspoon nutmeg

1 cup toasted walnuts, chopped

Directions:

Preheat oven to 350 F.
Add carrots to a large pot of salted water. Cook for 15 minutes, or until tender; drain, cool, and mash.
Mix mashed carrots with the remaining ingredients, except the walnuts.
Transfer mixture to a 2-quart casserole dish. Spread walnuts evenly on top.
Bake for 30 minutes.

Grain-free Granola

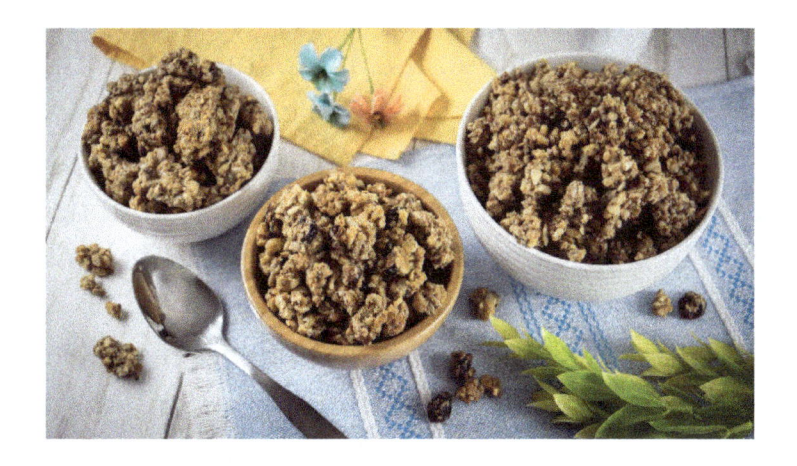

Cooking Time: 15 minutes
Servings: 2
Ingredients:

1 cup raw pecans
3/4 cup raw almonds
1/4 cup raw pumpkin seeds
1/4 cup raw unshelled sunflower seeds
1/4 cup unsweetened coconut flakes
1/2 cup raw honey
1/4 cup extra-virgin coconut oil
1/2 teaspoon ground cinnamon
1 teaspoon pure vanilla extract
1 cup dried cranberries
1 teaspoon unrefined sea salt

Directions:

Preheat oven to 270 F. Line a baking sheet with parchment paper.

Combine pecans, almonds, pumpkin seeds, sunflower seeds, and coconut flakes in a blender or food processor and process into smaller chunks.

Stir together the honey, coconut oil, cinnamon, and vanilla in a medium bowl and heat in the microwave for 30 seconds. Stir in the nut mixture.

Spread the mixture evenly onto the baking sheet. Bake mixture for about 20 minutes, or until lightly browned, stirring occasionally. Remove from oven and stir in the dried cranberries and salt.

Press mixture together until it forms a flat, smooth surface.

Let cool then cut into chunks.

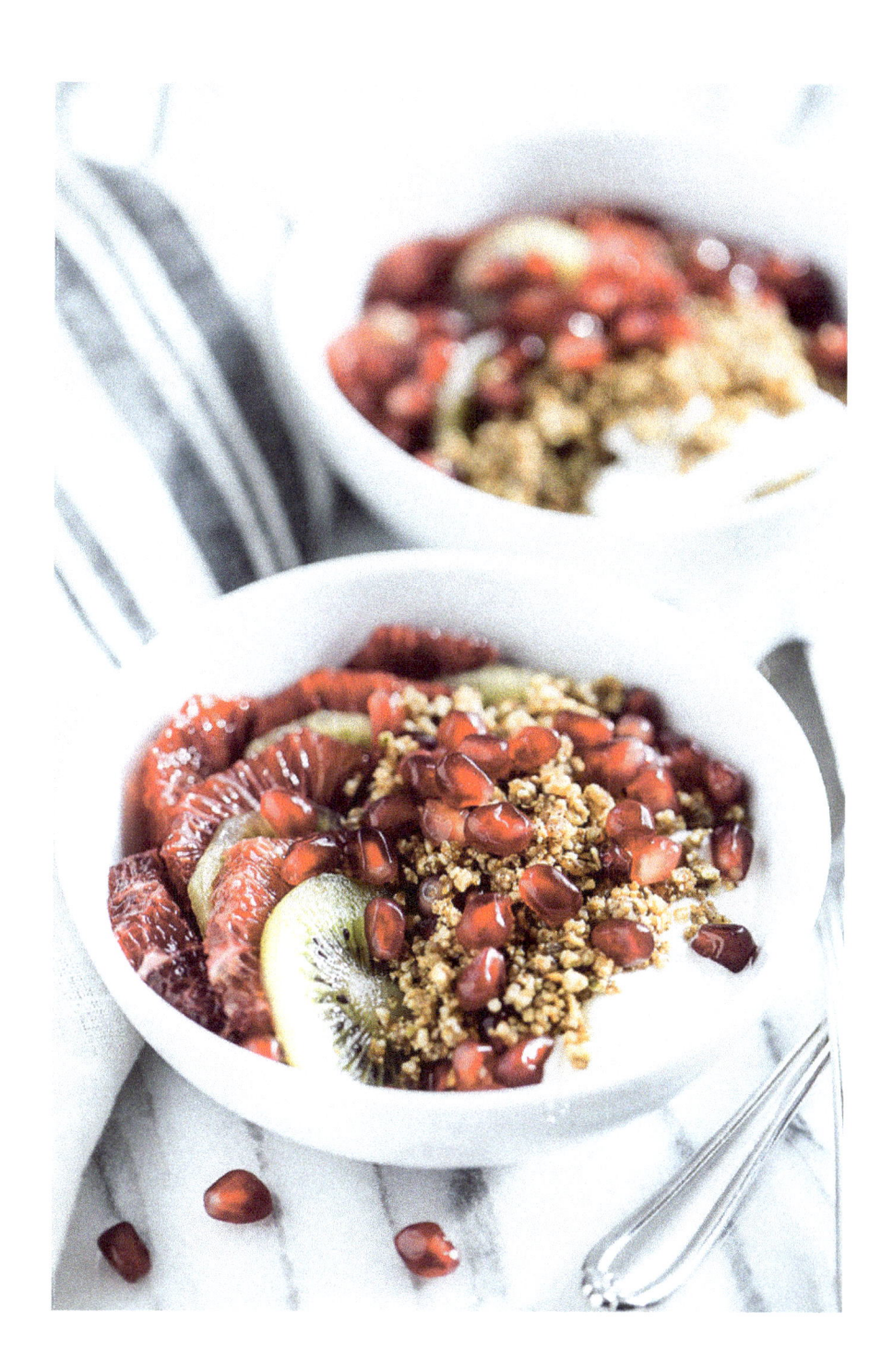

Conclusions

Breakfast is the most important meal of the day?

Absolutely yes, I hope you enjoyed this cookbook with an avalanche of recipes for breakfast, change often and take advantage of the variety of breakfasts that I have created for you.

Thank you very much for buying my book and I look forward to seeing you at the next cookbook. A big hug...

Erika Lombardi

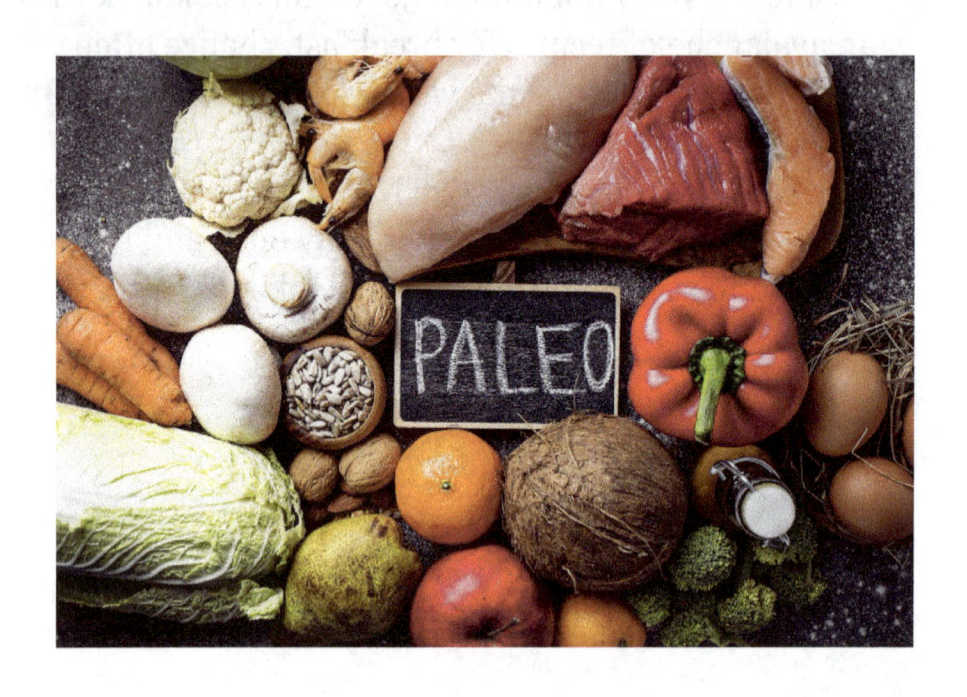

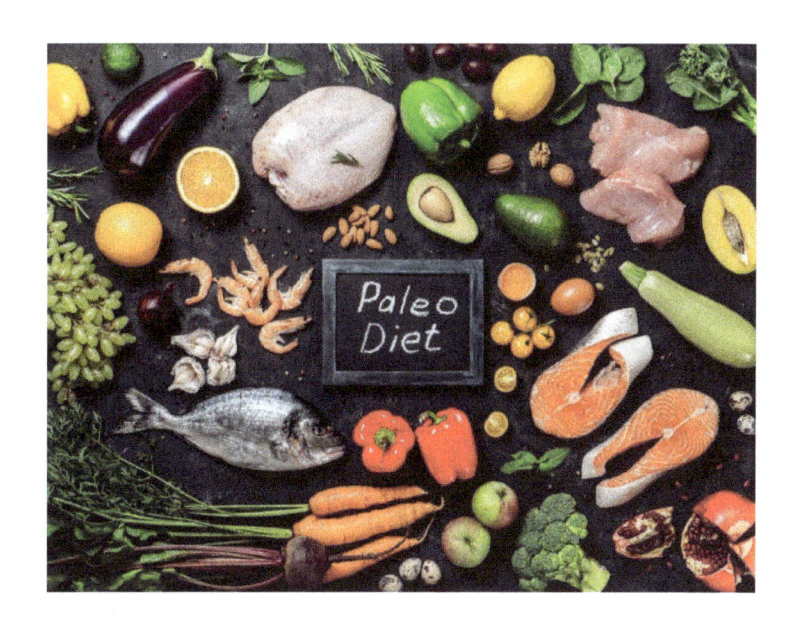

CPSIA information can be obtained
at www.ICGtesting.com
Printed in the USA
LVHW081607120621
690059LV00002B/206